Praise for *Strong Medicine*

"During a long and productive medical and academic career, Dr. Reece never lost his capacity for outrage at injustice and corruption. In *Strong Medicine,* he summons Dr. Tom Barrett and other people we learned to care about in his last novel, *Double Blind Double Cross,* to embody and express his outrage at the wrongdoing of so much of Big Pharma, to prove the enormity of the consequences of the wrongdoing, and to design a roadmap for correction. Dr. Reece tells an absorbing story, and, after reading it, it is impossible not to share his outrage."

—Judge Richard Cohen

"Once again, Bob Reece's passion for righting wrongs, sharing his love and skill in medical intrigue, and his deep knowledge and lifetime of experience as a compassionate physician, benefit us all as his dedicated readers. In these crazy times it can be hard to get into a book. But Bob has a talent of quickly capturing and keeping your attention. Tom is back and fighting his personal demons and the bad guys for all of us. Turn the page. It will be hard to stop reading till you get to the end."

—Lew Stern, PhD

"Dr. Robert Reece has the rare ability to create a fascinating fast-paced narrative anchored with clear technical description. Although a suspenseful novel, *Strong Medicine* is permeated with insights into modern healthcare and the pharmaceutical industry. Written in an intelligent way, but also a manner that the neophyte can understand, it is the story of an ideological doctor and his team on a quest to expose industry practices that cheat the individual or worse, encourage addiction to expensive drugs. In addition to the scientific aspect, it is also a nice story about finding love and the fundamental human relationships and needs we all have. Up to date with a nod to current politics and Covid, I very much enjoyed this book and look forward to Dr. Reece's next one.

—Kathryn Kleekamp

STRONG

MEDICINE

A Novel

ROBERT M. REECE, MD

Paperback ISBN: 978-0-9914-4242-3
Ebook ISBN: 978-0-9914424-3-0

Cover design by Thomas Tafuri

To patients everywhere who depend on prescribed medications to ease their symptoms and in some cases for their very survival.

The book is also dedicated to the thousands of ethical scientists and workers in the pharmaceutical industry whose work produces amazing drugs that alleviate human suffering.

Also by Robert M. Reece

About Ben

To Tell The Truth

Double Blind Double Cross

The Lewellyns from Vincennes

"Evil is like a shadow - it has no real substance of its own, it is simply a lack of light. You cannot cause a shadow to disappear by trying to fight it, stamp on it, by railing against it, or by any other form of emotional or physical resistance. In order to cause a shadow to disappear, you must shine a light on it."

—Shakti Gawain

CONTENTS

Introduction to the 2024 Edition

Some of the issues raised the previous edition of this book have been addressed during the Biden administration.

For example, the Inflation Reduction Act passed by Congress in 2022 put a cap of $35 per month out-of-pocket expense for insulin for Medicare recipients. President Biden called for this same cap (out-of-pocket cost of $35 per month) for all patients, regardless of insurance coverage, in his 2023 State of the Union address. Most drugmakers have since lowered the price of insulin to $35 per month with little loss to their profits, and building their public image.

Another major accomplishment of the Inflation Reduction Act relating to drug pricing was that Medicare can now negotiate with the pharmaceutical companies for the prices of ten selected drugs.

The savings to Medicare are considerable. (This information was adapted from CNN reports).

Prologue

Three Years Earlier

I arrived the same day as another doctor. Blond, blue-eyed and athletic, his rangy limbs and tanned craggy features cried out

"Surfer!"

"Hi. Tom Barrett," I said, extending my hand.

"Name's Danny Mott. You're the other surgeon, right?"

"Yep. First time deployed?"

"Yes. You?"

"Me too."

"You as tired as I am from the trip? Think we have time for a beer?" Danny asked.

"Yeah, I'm pooped. A beer sounds great. We're not on the schedule until tomorrow."

Soon our talk moved into our personal lives. Unlike me, he was married with a couple of boys, two and four years old.

"Here's Katharine," he said, passing his phone to me with videos of his wife. "She's a marine biologist at Scripps in La Jolla." In her wetsuit, she could have been an advertisement for health food as she toted her board toward the Pacific surf.

"And get these two guys. Lucky for them they look more like their mother than me. The four-year old here is

Hunter, named after Katharine's father. The little guy is two-year-old Jeff."

In the days to come I found Danny to be a splendid surgeon, steady, eager, and energetic. We worked together as though we'd been operating side-by-side for years. Outside the operating room we spent the little free time we had talking about life back home. We jogged around the camp when we could squeeze it in. Confiding in each other was natural.

"I'm a lucky guy, ya know," he told me after we stripped off our scrubs and got into our running gear. "Katharine's a woman in full. She's beautiful, sexy, funny as hell and a natural mother. The kids love playing soccer with her. You'll love her when you meet her."

I was sure when we got back to the States our friendship would flourish. Perhaps we would even team up professionally.

***

"Tom, I need you to help me check on a trooper in the helicopter before we move him," Major Higgins, our commanding officer, called out to me.

Christ, must be bad. The medics always brought the wounded directly into the operating theater. On our way out, we sidestepped a stretcher carrying a soldier, his bloody leg gaping from who knows what kind of shrapnel.

Just as Higgins and I got to the copter, BOOM! A deafening sound exploded from the operating station, not twenty yards away.

Oh my God! I froze. Looked at Higgins, who stared back, wide-eyed. Time did that weird thing where it stretches and detaches from its typical rhythm. We tore back to the unit.

I slid and nearly fell when I ran into what, mere moments before, had been the operating room. "Holy mother of…" I screamed. I was sliding on their guts, Danny's or the nurses' or from that poor guy on the stretcher. My puke was mixed with blood and flesh fragments on the floor or sprayed on the pocked walls. I retched my way beyond the blasted area, gasping for air.

After the acute horror and disbelief subsided turning into numb reality, Higgins gathered us together. He offered a short prayer and took a deep breath.

"This is devastating for all of us," he said in a practically inaudible voice. "We've lost five exemplary professionals, members of our team. Unbearable to contemplate the grief in their families, their wives, husbands, sons and daughters, parents and grandparents. What we do know is they'll suffer more than we." His voice broke and he sighed, standing up straighter as he continued. "A light's gone off in our spirit, but we have no choice but to press on."

Chapter 1

On the flight to San Diego, the rapid pulsations in Tom's ears were not from altitude, his eye blinking tears away not from dry cabin air. He shouldn't have chosen a seat so close to the engine. Its vibration and loud rumble triggered memory of that hideous day three years ago in Iraq when Danny Mott, his soul brother and surgical colleague, died from an improvised explosive device strapped to an enemy's body. The visuals were sharper now than when it happened. He felt suspended above that decimated operating room, looking down on the torn and shattered bodies of Danny and his nurse colleagues who lay dead, odors of blood and guts gathering in his olfactory hallucination.

Okay, he told himself, *breathe in, count to four, hold breath for seven, exhale eight.* After three rounds of breathing like that he felt his body relaxing. Maybe his underarm sweating was because he would soon see Katharine, Danny's widow? This was his second attempt to fulfill his promise to Danny to take care of her should anything happen to him. Tom had scoffed at the notion that anything would befall either of them, a huge dose of hope pushing down reality amid war's carnage.

Awkward was the only way to describe his last visit with Katharine. Full of embarrassing pauses, neither knew what purpose it was supposed to serve. The indifference shown him by Hunter and Jeff, her six- and four-year-old boys, was disconcerting but upon reflection, what could he expect from kids who didn't know him? They were only told that he was a good friend of their dead father.

His approaching rendezvous gave rise to troubling questions. What would they talk about? Their only common ground was Danny, and he was certain that Katharine didn't want to dwell on that heartache. He was also damned sure he didn't want to revisit Danny's horrible death, the fountainhead of his post-traumatic depression.

"Let's meet at my favorite restaurant in Del Mar," Katharine had suggested, remembering their mutual discomfort with Hunter and Jeff hanging around. "Name is 'The Fin,' mostly seafood, as you'd guess. No reservations and sometimes crowded but we can find a table in a corner."

Seems like a long ride from the airport to Del Mar. Tom's driver inundated him with a running travelogue of local landmarks.

"Thanks for all the information, but I need some quiet. How much further do we have to go?" Tom asked.

"Just a few more miles. Oh, oh, look out to your left, and you'll get a peek at the ocean."

Ten minutes later, they'd arrived. "How much do I owe you?"

"Uh, let's see. That's $37.00 altogether. Including tip."

Tom jumped out of the car with apprehension. He looked around, saw Katharine in line, and caught up with her.

"You found me!" she cried out. "Great. Cut in line here. You don't mind, do you?" she said and smiled at the man behind her.

The fellow didn't mind accommodating this beautiful woman. With glistening long brown hair with a stripe of gray at her forehead, large brown eyes, and a body like an exercise ad, she radiated charm. Katherine looked exactly like the pictures Danny had shown him when they were between operations in the military hospital. Before Danny was blown to bits.

They found a table next to a large picture window with a spectacular panorama of the Pacific. Lights played on the ocean where a few straggling die-hard surfers tried to catch a good wave.

"You ever surf here?" Tom asked, looking for safe conversational ground.

"Not the best place. It's better further north, around Cardiff. Do you surf?" she said with great interest. A second later, her face turned red when she realized what she'd forgotten. "Oh boy," she said, looking at Tom's paralyzed left arm. "Ew, dumb question. So sorry."

Tom's left arm was functionless due to injuries from a near-fatal assault. During his participation in a drug trial for post-traumatic stress disorder, he and another patient had discovered a competing pharmaceutical company had replaced the active drugs they were taking with sugar pills to sabotage the experiment. They were close to disclosing this when the competing company hired thugs to put a stop to their curiosity. At six feet-two, he was otherwise in excellent physical condition. His hairline was receding but a generous supply of brown, wavy hair remained. His eyes were radiantly blue, and his square jaw suggested determination and strength. He smiled easily, making movie-star good looks even more attractive.

"No problem. Never surfed, even before the arm thing. Grew up in Cincinnati where waterskiing on the Ohio River was the closest thing to surfing." *Would they ever get past awkwardness?*

"So, how are Jeff and Hunter?"

"Jeff is doing great. Remember, he hardly knew Danny, being so young when Danny went off to war. It probably affects me more than him that he won't know his father. Hunter, though, still has nightmares He's having a much harder time. He asks to see pictures of his father and wants to be reminded of their time together." Her face was drawn as she spoke of the children, but she forced a smile, apparently fighting off enveloping sadness. "Going into first grade soon. I'm hoping he'll get interested in his classmates and school and get past this."

She turned her attention to the menu, stopping the flow of conversation. They both ordered mahi mahi, neither knowing what to say while they waited for their food.

"How are you getting along?" Katharine asked, looking up from her plate once they'd been served.

"Very well, thanks," Tom replied, more stiffly than he intended. "I miss surgery, but my new non-profit gives me a sense of purpose. A lot to do getting it set up and running. I'm going to San Francisco tomorrow to see Amitav Kumar, a great guy who runs a non-governmental organization looking at corporate fraud. I'm looking forward to his advice about how to make this non-profit work."

Another uncomfortable lull magnified restaurant sounds and conversations from other tables. Tom had never been a talkative sort, and this uneasy meeting exacerbated his reticence. Katharine sensed his discomfort and reached across the table, placing her hand on his sleeve.

"We don't know each other very well, Tom. Tell me a little bit about yourself."

Tom flushed. He scratched his head, an old nervous habit and looked up at the ceiling while he offered the briefest of resumes.

"Well, grew up and went to college and medical school in Cincinnati, residency in surgery at Boston Medical Center, then to the Middle East War. That's about it." *What should I say about my time in the war? Talk about Danny?*

"That's when you met Danny, right?" So, Katharine brought it up.

Tom looked directly at her. She was staring back, trying not to betray emotions on her face. A wrinkled brow was an unmistakable giveaway.

"Uh, yeah." He looked down, then out to the ocean. He didn't want her to see tears forming as he thought of his deep friendship with Danny Mott. Working with that talented trauma surgeon had been the only joy within their hell, from the moment they met when he arrived.

But he couldn't tell Katharine his recurring flashback of the deafening explosion in the operating station with Danny and the nurses inside, killed instantly.

"Then you came back to Massachusetts?" Katherine asked, pulling him back to the present.

"Uh huh." *Should I tell her about what happened with Laxalta?*

"Were you injured in the war, or did you go back to doing surgery?" she asked.

"Well, no." *What should he tell this virtual stranger who happened to be the wife of his soul mate in war?* As he looked at her sympathetic face, he decided to tell her about his PTSD diagnosis, the drug trial at the Zylinski Institute, his abduction, and beating – the whole thing. He hadn't talked to anyone outside of his therapy cocoon about these things.

"How terrible for you," Katherine said as she absorbed his words. "Bad enough that you have post-traumatic stress, but to go through all of that."

"Well, it's over now," he said, not wanting their time to dissolve into a pity party. "What went on in that drug trial opened my eyes to the inside of the drug industry. Not all companies, of course. Most drug makers are supplying needed drugs at reasonable prices to consumers, but the public needs to be shown what some rogue companies are doing."

"What's next?" Katharine asked.

"Have PharmaTruth, my new non-profit organization, be the vehicle to uncover examples of unethical behavior. I'm anxious to see where I can go with this."

"That's a great name, but sorry, I'm a little confused. Tell me what PharmaTruth is supposed to do."

Tom, happy to be on familiar ground, replied with his "elevator pitch."

"Expose greedy practices in the pharmaceutical industry; spotlight price gouging, promotional schemes to induce doctors, nurses and other health providers to prescribe certain drugs; confusing advertising; suppression of competition by generic drugs. I hope by unmasking bad practices we can ensure necessary drugs are in reach of those who need them."

"Wow. Good stuff. I love it. Every time I go for my prescriptions or ones for the boys, I'm blown away by how expensive they are. My insurance covers most of my costs, but for people with inadequate insurance, it must be so frustrating. I can't imagine having to choose between eating or filling a prescription."

Katharine was intrigued by Tom's story. "So where did this 'Change the World' drive come from? Your family? Are they still in Cincinnati?"

"No, both dead. Years ago."

"Oh. I'm so sorry. Do you have brothers, sisters…cousins?"

"Nope. None of those either."

Hearing how isolated he was, kindled Katherine's caretaker instincts.

"So, where did your Don Quixote bent come from?" she said.

"I guess both Mom and Dad. They were decent people, tried to do the right thing."

Katharine waited for him to describe his parents further, but when nothing else was forthcoming, she asked, "Do you have friends in Boston?"

"Mostly professional friends, people who saw me through the months at Zylinski and the clinical trial." Tom realized he'd been tumbling from one phase of life to the next with no time for reflection. He couldn't think of anyone he'd call to have a beer or go to a concert or a movie with. The sound of the surf outside induced a wave of loneliness that washed over him.

Katharine saw he was lost in thought, paused a few moments, then said in a low voice, "You sound kinda alone."

"Huh? Oh. Yep, guess I am."

"You have a lot of heart for someone alone in the world." Katharine smiled at him.

It's getting as easy to talk honestly with her as it was with Danny. Should I tell her about Cynthia? He decided to forge ahead. He'd gone this far, might as well get it all out.

"I broke up recently with a woman I lived with for four years before the war. When I came back, it didn't work out." Tom stopped short of opening up further. "I haven't really been in the market for—-what's the term now? --a 'significant other.' Preoccupied with PharmaTruth, working on that full time.

"How are *you* doing?" Tom asked, trying to get out of the spotlight. But as soon as his words floated across the table, he saw tears gather.

"Well, therapy helps," she said. "And exercise, mainly surfing." She raised her glass to her lips and sipped the cool wine. "You know, it's interesting how easy it is talking with you. I hardly know you. I can't get into it with friends or coworkers. But Danny told me in his letters that you were such a kind, good man; so, I feel I can trust you."

"Kind and good," Tom snorted. "I used to think I was both, but that was before the war. When I came back from the Middle East, I was so angry, confused and out of control, I did things…well…" He searched for words. "Things I'm sorry about. When the world does a number on you, thrusting you into war, or poverty, or into some other kind of injustice, you get scared and lash out. I guess that's how we all get when we're fighting for survival. Until I got treated, I was ready to explode.

"But I can't imagine what it's like for you," he said. "I knew Danny for only a few weeks and thought he'd be a life-long friend. We had so much in common. But you, God, he was your husband, the father of your kids. That's a whole different order of love."

Katharine's jaw muscles were taut, and a look of firmness came over her face as she watched the waves breaking over a jetty.

"I've got to stay strong for the boys," she said. "If they catch me crying or looking the least bit morose, they react to it with hyperactivity and fighting. I have to hide my feelings. But yes, it's intense; I miss Danny every day." Tears dropped onto her plate. She took a deep breath, wiped her face with her napkin. "Sorry, I promised myself I wouldn't do this."

"Please, don't apologize. You're entitled."

Katharine looked out again at the ocean, then turned back to Tom.

"In my dreams, he's still alive. He walks through our door, hugs me, the kids jump all over him, rolling around in raucous laughter. I can't erase this dream. It comes every night, wakes me up. Getting back to sleep is impossible. I'm always tired, just putting one foot in front of the other most of the time." Katharine folded her napkin, placed it neatly on the table. "It doesn't seem real that Danny is dead. Remains were sent to me to bury or cremate, but a container with God-knows-what inside did nothing to convince me, nothing concrete to tell me in absolute terms that he was actually dead. No way of bringing a sense of closure to this awful thing. I don't even know where he died. Sure, I know it was in some godforsaken sandy place in the Middle East desert, but it's not a real place in the world. You know how people put up crosses on the sides of highways where their loved ones died in an auto crash? I don't even have that satisfaction." She dried her eyes and looked away from Tom, the moment drawn out.

Tom pondered how to address convincing Katharine that Danny was indeed dead. Not a subject to be dealt with easily. He'd come back to that later.

"Work?" Tom said finally, looking for a safe space.

"Going well," she said, relieved the tension was broken. "My boss is patient and understanding. Work is therapeutic. It's where I can get lost."

"What do you do?"

"I work on the squid axon. Sounds boring, but really it isn't," she said.

Tom laughed.

"Sorry, don't mean to be defensive, but most people yawn when I tell them that."

"I'm pretty sure I know some people in Woods Hole doing similar work, so I'm not laughing at your work. It was cute you were standing up for the squid." Tom smiled at her and she relaxed.

"My co-workers are sympathetic and supportive, but I wish they'd be their old selves, sarcastic and teasing, giving me a hard time about little things. Kidding around. That doesn't happen anymore. They see me now as a fragile creature, about to collapse at the least little comment."

"People seldom know how to empathize without feeling they're being patronizing," Tom said. "Ever try writing a sympathy note? You try to express support, avoiding clichés like 'thoughts and prayers are with you.' Worst is the Pollyanna who says stupid things like 'time heals all wounds' or 'give it some time and it'll be okay' or 'women are better at these losses than men' (usually from a well-meaning man). The only thing time may do is allow us to carve out coping skills. And not everyone does that." *Oh, boy, enough sadness, time to lighten up.* Tom smiled and poured each another glass of wine.

"So, I told you about myself; how about you?"

She smiled. "Well, born in Boulder, where my parents still live. Dad loves to ski. Mom is a sculptress, pretty good, has her own studio. One older brother Howie, three years older than I, so about 39. We don't see each other much. He lives in Singapore, in business, married, no kids. That's about it."

She looked at her watch and gasped.

"I gotta go! My sitter needs to get home. I'm already late." She pulled out her phone, sent a quick text, and said, "Where are you staying? Can I drop you off?"

"No, thanks for the offer. Got a room at the hotel near the airport. Early flight tomorrow to San Francisco. I'll get an Uber."

Katharine laughed, looking even more lovely than the pictures Danny had shown him. He was sure other men noticed her, how could they not?

They stood looking at each other, neither knowing what to do. Finally, she moved in for a hug and Tom wrapped his good right arm around her waist.

"Stay in touch," Katherine said, disengaging. "I'm so gla to talk with you. It's rare that I can unload with so much freedom. I appreciate your understanding."

"So good to see you. Say hello to the boys, even though they may not remember me," Tom said.

"Oh, they remember you. They've talked about you and were disappointed they weren't coming tonight. I told them we needed to talk about grown-up stuff. They complained, but they like the sitter, so they're fine." She waved and was off.

Tom watched as she slid into her car and sped away. Her fragrance, her essence filled his consciousness. The stirring in his groin signaled his arousal, surprising him. Confused, he shook his head and scheduled a ride.

***

Katharine peeled out of The Fin's parking lot. Her phone chimed and the speaker in the car picked up Barry Ringer's voice.

"Hey Kath, where are you? Missed seeing you at the going away party for Roger."

"Oh, sorry about that. I had a dinner meeting with a friend in Del Mar. Just heading home. How was the party?"

"As you'd imagine; everyone saying nice things about Rog, toasts, that kind of thing. You know he's headed to MBL in Woods Hole, right? Don't envy him going from our wonderful climate to frigid New England weather. But he seems happy.

"When am I going to see you?" he asked.

"Well, not tonight," Katharine said as she pulled into her carport. "I'm already late for the sitter and the boys will need my attention."

"Okay, I'll talk to you later," he said in his low baritone. "Love you."

"Okay. Maybe tomorrow. Bye," she said.

They'd been seeing each other for about six months. It was a pleasant, but not exciting, relationship. Working together at Scripps had been the platform for their friendship before Barry's divorce, and their bond had evolved to some degree, once he was, in his words, "a free man." He was warm and comfortable and intellectually her equal. She enjoyed his company. He was even a pretty good surfer. But still…

"Lisa, I'm home! Sorry to be so late. Everything okay?" she called as she hurried into the house.

"No problem, we're fine," Lisa said. "They're in their PJ's."

"I'm sick!" Hunter groaned. "Where've you been?"

"Me too!" whined Jeff.

"They're not either, they're just trying to make you feel guilty. Be quiet, you two and give your mother a hug," Lisa said with a wide grin.

But as usual, they *were* successful making her feel guilty. She was their only parent, what if something happened to her when she was out? A car accident, a shooting? Ugh. But how would they ever have a father if she didn't date? Not that tonight was a date. Oh boy, crying over Danny. Not a way to show a handsome man that even in her grief, she was still open to the possibility of love. Complicated, to say the least. Though she kind of felt a vibe. Tom's probably too loyal to Danny to even consider it, she thought, and went off to tuck in the males who currently occupied her heart.

Chapter 2

Tom's thoughts bounced between Katharine and the upcoming visit in San Francisco with Amitav Kumar, a mentor on creating watchdog organizations. He could almost smell Katharine's perfume, see her eyes, feel her presence. She'd had a dizzying effect on him, and he was emotionally off-balance from their meeting. Despite this, he managed to find his way to Kumar's office in a high-rise building with a view of Coit Tower.

From the moment Tom stepped into the lobby of Amitav Kumar's offices he felt he was under surveillance. What Tom was about to launch could put him once more into the crosshairs of danger from powerful forces, a situation he'd barely survived before. How many near misses does a man have? He'd lost function in his left arm in that fracas. What lay ahead in this new battle?

"So, since our quick meeting last time, what's happening?" Kumar asked once Tom was seated in his office.

"Quite a bit, but still trying to pull my ideas together. Hope you can help me sort a few things out."

Tom glanced at Kumar's desk and a brass-framed picture of who must be his wife and two kids. He wondered how old they were, how recent the picture was. His wife, a gorgeous Indian woman, appeared about thirty-five. Considering Kumar looked to be in his mid-fifties, Tom wondered if this was an old picture or if he simply had a young wife.

"Well, you told me you have a board and mission statement. Non-profit 101," Kumar said. "Running my place here to expose corporate fraud has taught me some hard-won lessons," Kumar sighed. "I wonder if you might be having any second thoughts. I know you were a doc in the war. Sure you don't want a more relaxing second career?"

"What happened to me after I got back from the war changed me in several ways. It made me furious that a pharmaceutical corporation would almost kill me to protect their profits, so my instinct is revenge. I'm also discovering that what that company did to sabotage the clinical trial I was in might be a cultural norm in the industry.

"But I want to hear about is your experience in taking on powerful and possibly ruthless adversaries. And don't leave out advice on how to avoid getting badly hurt," Tom said, grinning.

Kumar sat forward and placed his folded hands on his desktop.

"Rule Number One: don't expect too much too soon. Start slowly, follow up on all plausible leads, but be damned careful," he said. "There are people who don't want anything to rock their yachts. Watching your back is a 24-hour necessity.

"On the other hand, the second rule is to not see evil everywhere. Most companies try to do the right thing, even though the bottom line is their guiding star. Pick those with the most egregious practices to expose."

"Yeah, I'm researching companies, but figuring out which ones are the dirtiest isn't easy. There is a huge lack of transparency. News accounts help, but they're variable in their credibility. There are already other small groups of people trying to expose bad behaviors, but their findings are published in obscure places and they do a lot of preaching to the choir. Any suggestions on how to get information not typically put into the public domain?"

"It's more and more difficult with social media making so much unfiltered content and bad information available. So much of it is opinion, biased, politically driven, or just plain fraudulent. This means you must research meticulously. Don't go off half-cocked. Doing that ends in no gain and possible disaster. When I started out, I made a lot of mistakes, but luckily none was crippling." Kumar paused, gazed out the window, trying to decide how best to advise Tom. "What is your major worry at this point?"

"Well, your warning about not going off half-cocked is one of my concerns. I have PTSD, under pretty good medical control, but I still get real pissed off when I see injustice."

"That sense of injustice can be used for good. But keep your cool. Don't come off as angry or belligerent even though that's in style these days. That will pass, I hope, as people tire of bluster and nastiness. Stay adult, rational, and open-minded, but not so open that your brains fall out." He smiled, then continued.

"The sad reality is that facts or appeals to angels and their better nature never convince people frozen in their beliefs. They'll go down in flames rather than admit they're wrong. Most people are frightened and insecure, protecting their self-interest above all else.

"I guess, lastly, but vitally, is to be wary of whom to trust."

"Oh, I've learned that the hard way," Tom said. "You asked about my worries. Well one major worry is just that—who to trust. I confided in one of my doctors in my treatment program at Zylinski. He betrayed me and I ended up in the back of a van headed for a warehouse where I was beaten to a pulp."

"That's a gruesome story. But you learned an important lesson, that trusting others is tricky. Confide in perhaps two or three people. That caution shouldn't translate into paranoia, but it means remaining circumspect about sharing your thoughts and feelings. And of course, putting security measures in place."

Before Tom could ask about providing security, and whether he *had* been scrutinized when he entered the building, Kumar's phone rang. As Kumar excused himself to answer, Tom couldn't help admiring this benign-appearing man. Greying hair and a diminutive frame belied his inner intensity and steeliness. He exuded confidence laced with a big helping of humility. *Was this part of his Hindu culture?* Tom's curiosity overcame his innate disinclination to pry into the evolution of his convictions. When Kumar finished his call, Tom asked, "Pardon my nosiness, but how'd you get in this work?"

Kumar chuckled. "It's a familiar story around Silicon Valley. After college, about thirty years ago, I went to work with a startup computer chipmaker in San Jose. Started out as a chemist burning chips, then promotions came quickly."

"What company was that?" Tom asked.

"This little place bloomed into the behemoth that's now called Intel. I took all stock options they offered and bought more on my own. I invested most of my salary in the company. Stocks soared so I retired when I was fifty with a huge nest egg. That golden little egg has only grown."

"You could have gone to Hawaii for the rest of your life."

Kumar laughed. "In truth, I considered that. I'd been going to Hanalei on holiday for several years and love it there. But after about a year of no purpose, other than hedonism, I got bored, wondered what I should do with my life."

"How did you decide to pursue revealing corporate wrongdoing?"

"I'd seen a lot of shady stuff in the tech world, not at Intel, but other companies. Ambitious young guys who'd do most anything to make a buck. Growing up in India, I'd always been taught to be honest. Then, my brother got swept up in a company's misdeeds and he ended up taking the blame and doing jail time for some of the upper echelon people who went unscathed. I thought someone needs to expose fraudulent behavior, so it might as well be me. It's become my raison d'être."

"Family?"

"Yes." Kumar smiled widely. "A wonderful wife—a gynecologist—two adult children, scientists: an astrophysicist and a solar engineer. We live quietly in Marin County in a small home with all kinds of security devices. One can't be too careful."

"So that picture on your desk is a little dated?"

"Oh yeah, maybe 15 years old. My wife looks the same, still beautiful, still wonderful. But the kids are grown and on their own. I miss them."

Kumar's phone rang again. "Yeah, OK. Thanks.

"Sorry, need to run to a meeting," he said rising to shake Tom's hand. "What are you doing for dinner?"

"No plans. Headed home in the morning so I'll probably catch a bite and turn in early."

"Do you like Indian cuisine? We could have dinner together at a great restaurant, about a block from here. My wife is on call tonight so I won't see her probably until tomorrow."

"Wonderful!" Tom said, flattered and happy that he'd get to spend more time with Kumar.

***

It was clear by how they were greeted that Kumar ate at the Curry Leaf often. They were shown to their table and tea was brought as soon as they were seated.

Tom took in the darkly lit décor. Suddenly goosebumps prickled his neck. *Hold on. Wasn't that guy over there hanging around the reception desk at Kumar's office? He's huge.*

"My bodyguard," Kumar said, noticing Tom and his furrowed brow as he stared at this fellow.

"Oh. Wow. Pretty serious security measures," Tom said. His rapid heartbeat slowed down, and he deferred to Kumar when ordering. After the waitress left, Kumar set his teacup down.

"Tom," Kumar said. "Tell me more about how you got interested in smoking out the bad guys."

"It's complicated," Tom said with his usual hesitancy to open up. "I certainly didn't go to medical school to run a non-profit. But as you've surely noticed, my left arm is paralyzed. My surgical career evaporated."

Kumar leaned forward. "My wife would be spiritless without performing surgery. A loss like that must be terribly painful. How did it happen, if you don't mind my asking?"

Tom took a deep breath and looked up from the plate of food that had been served. Kumar was studying his face intently. But Tom felt his empathy.

"When I got back from the Middle East War with PTSD, I entered a drug research trial run by my friend and former surgical colleague, Akira Yamaguchi. In the study, patients' initial improvements were followed by a sudden relapse of their PTSD symptoms."

Tom's mouth went dry as he recalled those dark days. He sipped some tea and looked at Kumar.

"Sorry, I have trouble talking about this. Brings back some awful memories."

"We can skip it. I want this to be a pleasant meal for you," Kumar said.

"No," Tom said. "I think telling you may be therapeutic." He paused, pushed his chair back from the table, ran his fingers through his hair. "Anyhow, Akira asked me to help him figure out what was going wrong." Tom spooled out the rest of his story to Amitav's astonishment.

Kumar was shaking his head and rolling his eyes.

"I thought *I* was dealing with bad actors. That's really disgusting."

"It gets much worse, but I won't tell you the details. Sometimes it seems remote. Another lifetime. But it really wasn't that long ago, which I guess is why it still gets me heated."

"Can take years to get over trauma," Kumar said. "That's how your arm got paralyzed?"

"Yeah. I got a big legal settlement for my efforts. While I was rehabbing, I had plenty of time to read about big pharma. The more I read, the more I was convinced there needed to be an expose of this industry. Some of them were behaving badly, to say the least."

Kumar sighed. "Really similar to my motivation. I can't tell you how glad I am knowing you're doing this. Whatever help I can give you is yours. Just ask."

"Well, I don't want to be vulnerable again, so I might need the number for Bodyguards Unlimited," Tom said, looking over at the burly guy a couple tables away.

And the risks he was about to take finally sunk in.

Chapter 3

Reginald Warner tossed his empty cigarette pack into a waste can in his private lavatory at Pylea Pharmaceuticals. He looked in the mirror to check on his aging process. His head was smooth with no grooves or depressions -- or hair. His ears had become larger and more prominent as he'd grown older. Before he lost his hair, it was black, but after a melanoma was excised from his nose, chemotherapy denuded his scalp and saved his life. His hair never grew back. His left eyelid had always drooped, the result of a birth injury. Despite this, he thought, not bad for a sixty-seven-year-old guy.

His orthopedist advised him his arthritic limp would be remedied easily with a hip replacement, but Warner told the doctor to go to hell. Not a man to mince words, his colorful language was legendary in the drug industry, as were his dalliances.

"The meeting with that doctor from Hempstead. Is it set for next Tuesday?" he asked Roy Shelby, his secretary.

"At two. He's bringing a guy with him, not sure what his role is."

"A lawyer?"

"He didn't say."

"Maybe we ought to get Bernie to sit in on the meeting. Can't be too careful."

"I'll tell him to be here. It's just a preliminary meeting, you know. No papers to sign, no contracts, any of that stuff."

"The recording apparatus is all set up though?"

"Yep, just as you ordered."

"I got psyched when I heard about this new antibiotic. It could make my company millions of dollars if we play our cards right. I know how to play those cards, too. It's not for nothing I spent all those years in Texas learning the ropes. This drug will be in such high demand every hospital will be drooling over it. We can make a killing, all in the name of helping patients. But we gotta be careful. I don't know much about this doctor coming to see us. He could be trouble. We'll have to keep our guard up.

Chapter 4

Getting through airport security isn't easy when your left arm is hanging loose at your side. Once aboard, Tom struggled to hoist his carry-on into the overhead, vainly refusing help from a strong-looking woman. Finally, he was strapped in his seat with plenty of time for contemplation ahead.

Could a relationship with the widow of a guy that felt like my brother ever bloom into anything more than platonic friendship? Do I want it to? Sure felt like there was potential. For the first time in months, I felt a flicker of sexual tension, so I'm definitely physically attracted to her. But will the phantom of Danny always float over us? Will Danny become more idealized as his death becomes more distant? What about Hunter and Jeff? And for chrissake, she lives three thousand miles away! Just forget about it. It's impractical, too emotionally complicated. And after losing a paragon like Danny, she's probably not even interested in romance with anyone else. Or if she does have human impulses, maybe she already has someone. She didn't seem open to a man in her life, but who knows?

Tom hadn't slept well at the hotel, too much buzzing in his head and party noise in the hall. He put on his headphones and after the plane leveled off, he slipped easily into sleep. Still groggy when he got off the plane, he slept again when he was in his own bed.

***

The next morning, Tom woke up to startling numbers on his clock. *What the…ten o'clock? Shit, board meeting at eleven! First meeting of this terrific new group of people. I have to introduce board members to each other, get them psyched up. A pivotal day for PharmaTruth and I'm already running late.* He jumped out of bed, threw on some clothes, and ran to the office on Mt. Vernon Street. At least he'd made a good decision to live in a condo close by on Joy Street.

"Well Dr. Barrett, so glad you could make it!" Dolores said with her hand on her hip, a tilt of her head and eyes that showed mock impatience with her new boss. Dolores Whitcomb, a Black woman old enough to be Tom's mother (and who acted like she was his mother), took Tom by his good arm and led him into his office. The new board was assembling in the conference room down the hall.

"You trying to give me a heart attack?" she chided.

"Sorry, got back from California late last night. Crashed at home and forgot the alarm. What have you cooked up for the meeting?"

"Well, all those suits are waiting in there for marching orders. Here's the agenda. Say hello and ask folks to introduce themselves. Be sure to say they should limit themselves to 25 words or less or who knows when you'll get to your mission statement slash rousing speech to coalesce the troops.

"Thanks, Dolores," he said sheepishly. They walked into a large conference room where new board members and three staff were taking their seats. Conversation was at a high pitch.

"Morning everyone, please take a seat. I'm Tom Barrett," he shouted over the din. "You've already met my assistant, Dolores Whitcomb." The chatter dissipated as all heads turned toward him. "Although I founded this organization, you, the board, will shape and guide it. Thank you all for coming."

Tom scanned the table. He'd had a lot of help identifying and recruiting top-notch people. All were between forty and sixty years of age. Five were women, including one Black psychologist, an Asian businesswoman, one Latino community representative, a woman journalist, and the rest were men: three physicians, a pharmacist, a pharmacologist, an economist and two businessmen. He was proud he'd been able to persuade them all to join as unpaid board members.

"This organization has a golden opportunity to force big pharma to fulfill their obligation to provide their product more fairly to people, not only in this country but around the world. For too long drugs have been out of reach for many who need them because of cost barriers or by inaccessibility. PharmaTruth aims to change that dramatically and it is way past due!

"Since this is a non-profit organization, some of you may wonder if one of your jobs is to raise money, the central objective of most non-profit board members. The old story is 'give or get.' That expectation doesn't apply to PharmaTruth. I received a substantial legal financial settlement from a pharmaceutical company for their interference in a drug trial. This money provides operating funds for PharmaTruth for a long time. So, your job is to be our brain trust. When I look around this table, I sincerely marvel at the breadth and depth of your experience and knowledge. Your contributions will be to answer questions in your sphere of expertise. Our staff will assist you as we get underway."

Tom invited the board members to introduce themselves briefly as Dolores suggested. For some it was hard but after a few minutes the introductions were concluded, agreement was reached for a date for the next meeting, and they filed out, once again in a flurry of talk.

"Think we're off to a good start," Tom said to Delores, who nodded as they left the conference room.

***

Tom was staring out his window, mulling over last week's meeting when his phone rang.

"Dr. Barrett, Sebastian Arnhold here," one of his board members said. "I'm calling to suggest a guy for our board who used to work for the FDA, got frustrated with the Feds, and now works for the university where I teach. He's a pharmacologist, a great professor with terrific presentation skills. He's also got bureaucratic blood running in his veins. He knows how organizations work and how they fail. I think he could help us, sort of frame our mission and help us with strategy."

"Terrific!" Tom said. "Have you told him about us? If I call him, will he know why?"

"Yeah, I told him about our first board meeting. His name is Reed Burseik. He's pumped about getting involved. I'm emailing his name and contact information."

"I'll call him today. And thanks."

Just what we need. Tom had been in a haze since he started this venture, not sure how to proceed. This wasn't surgery. He had zero training and experience in the ways of corporations, profit or non-profit. He didn't waste any time. After he got past two administrative assistants, Tom began his pitch.

"Dr. Burseik, this is Tom Barrett from PharmaTruth. Sebastian Arnhold gave me your name and said you'd be a great person to help us get organized. I understand he told you what we're trying to do."

"Yeah, he gave me the broad outlines of your outfit. I'd like to be a part of this. How can I get involved?"

"I'd appreciate your coming to the next board meeting to facilitate discussion about what we should and shouldn't do. Tell us what kinds of roadblocks and resistance we'll face and how to anticipate and prepare for them."

"I'm eager to help," Burseik said. "Send me everything you've got about the structure, function, mission, and vision for your outfit. I'll rough out a presentation to get the juices flowing at the next meeting."

***

Board members straggled into the conference room, so it was 2:30 when the meeting started. Dolores gave each a handout as they walked in the doors. Tom was discreetly quiet until they had taken their seats and stillness descended on the room.

"Thank you all for coming," Tom began. "I have the pleasure of introducing Dr. Reed Burseik, formerly with the FDA, who will help focus our efforts." He told them some of Burseik's background and that he would be leading today's discussion.

In his mid-fifties, Burseik's gray hair and well-trimmed beard were accented by dark-rimmed glasses. His slender frame spoke of hours in the gym. His accent was nondescript, so Tom assumed he grew up in California or the Midwest.

"I looked over the ambitious goals Tom has set forth," Burseik said. "Reminds me of the Yiddish saying, 'Man plans, and God laughs.' This is further truth that God is a woman.

"Tom's list of culpable practices in the pharmaceutical industry is comprehensive, as you can see." Burseik nodded toward the handouts. "But addressing such an extensive list is probably not doable, frankly. We need to drill down, prioritize, and strategize about attacking those we can do something about."

The more Tom listened to the board members enthusiastically following Burseik's lead, the more he realized the problems they sought to address were deeper and wider than he imagined. He'd have to find at least two more analysts to refine data this project would generate.

After about forty-five minutes, Burseik looked at his watch.

"So, we've identified four major foci for our efforts. It's getting late and I'm going to toss these hot potatoes to Tom and his staff to work on." He glanced around the table. "Thanks for all your input. This has been a good exercise. See you next meeting."

Tom walked out behind Burseik and pulled him into his office.

"Thanks for a fantastic beginning," Tom said.

"It *was* a productive meeting," Reed said. "Lots of good ideas and a high passion level, higher than I expected for an early meeting of a new board. Now," he looked squarely into Tom's eyes, "your job is to keep that passion hot." He held him in his gaze for a moment. "Have a plan for that?"

Tom stared back at him, recalling a time when his surgical mentors nailed him with questions during an operation. His mind went vacant.

"As a matter of fact, no," he finally said and shrugged.

"I'm really excited by this," Burseik said. "I think I could help you develop strategy and keep the group fired up." He looked away for a moment. "I'm going to be rather brazen. I wonder, is there room in your budget for me as a consultant?"

Tom was surprised by this prospect. He liked what he'd seen of Burseik so far and didn't want to lose his help. He gave it some quick thought.

"There's room in the budget for people who can contribute. I've seen what you've already done for the board, and I like it. What do you have in mind?"

"I have a job, as you know, but I could consider being your operating officer on a half-time basis. The university allows for this kind of thing. My current grant is about to run out, so I'll have time in a couple of months."

"We can work out terms in my office," Tom exclaimed. "Let's sit down and talk turkey."

"You are a surgeon, after all," Burseik said. "Quick decisions. Let's do it!"

Chapter 5

After signing a contract, Burseik left. Tom tapped his pen on the desk, his left eyelid twitched. *Was I too impulsive? I'm the Founder and CEO: I can hire and fire staff. But what if the board gets disenchanted and thinks I acted inappropriately? It's* my *money that funds the place. But still, I should have consulted the board before signing Burseik.* He was feeling his way in an unfamiliar role. *Don't I need someone like Burseik to manage PharmaTruth?* Management knowledge was not part of his skill set and Burseik came highly recommended by Sebastian Arnhold, a board member about whom Tom knew – almost nothing. *But I must trust someone, right? That's what Kumar said.* After allowing his paranoia full rein, he got hold of himself and relaxed. Burseik was competent and equipped to manage, so Tom's fretting gradually subsided. *I need to learn to trust myself.*

He'd talk about it tonight when some of the board members were going for dinner at Luca's in the North End around seven. Tom checked his phone and saw a familiar phone number but couldn't remember whose it was. *Better call it now, could be important.*

"Hi, Tom Barrett returning your call."

"I know it's you, you lunkhead!" came the answer from a voice more recognizable than anyone's.

"Cynthia! How are you?" he shouted.

"Doing well. Working hard, trying to keep this nursing school afloat. Getting applicants is challenging. Too many young women going into medicine, law, business, physical therapy, even politics. Too few want the demands of nursing. And not enough males entering the field."

"You're sounding like a curmudgeon bemoaning 'kids today,'" Tom said, teasing her. "Seriously, though, it's all changing for sure. Medicine's now half women," he grumped, but then realized he was in dangerous waters. "But they're damned good from what I hear," he said, trying to run back from a dangerous precipice. "I'm too far removed from it all to know, really.

"So how are you otherwise?" he asked, changing the subject. *Is she married, or in love, or still avoiding a lasting relationship? Why in hell is she calling? She sounds like her old self, though, giving him a hard time.*

"Same. I'm so consumed with work I don't reflect on life much," she said. She, too, wondered if her ex had a significant other by now. He was a handsome dude and too sexy for his own good.

He paused, unsure of where the conversation was going.

"You still there?" Cynthia asked.

"Yeah, still here. Frankly, trying to figure out why you're calling," he ventured. With Cynthia it was always better to speak one's mind.

"I'd like to see you."

So typical of Cynthia, direct, straight to the point, no bullshit.

"I think of you a lot," she continued, "and wonder how you're doing. Maybe have dinner? Out, at a restaurant of your choice. You probably know all the latest and greatest restaurants in Boston. I'll come in and meet you someplace."

Tom looked at the ceiling, closed his eyes, and recalled their last time together when she said, "I can't lie to myself anymore; I can't give you what you need. I think we both need a fresh start."

"How long has it been since we've had dinner together?" he said, coming out of his reminiscences.

"Time enough to gain some perspective," she said in a soft voice. "What do you say?"

"Okay, an offer I can't refuse," he decided. "How about the Red Fez in the South End? They have the most authentic Middle Eastern food in Boston. I'm free tomorrow or Saturday."

"Let's do Saturday. Some of us work on Friday! Say about seven?"

"Great. See you there. And Cynthia?"

"Yes?"

"Wear that scarf, you know, the one with the Asian print?"

"Okay. Bye."

So now the door to that sealed-off room was ajar. *Why did I tell her what to wear?* Old feelings and memories floated out: their first date, dinner in her South End Warren Street condo, trips together before his military service. Idyllic times. All that changed when he returned from war and PTSD horrors erupted: nightmares and flashbacks, putting Cynthia at risk for bodily harm. Tom's pulse rose and his palms moistened as these images sprang out of dark recesses. He paced his office, glanced at the clock. Glad he was having dinner with new friends from his board. This would compel him to focus on present tense life. But recollections of those cherished times with Cynthia tarnished by his postwar deterioration crowded into his psyche as he walked the ten minutes to Luca's.

The North End had always held charms for Tom. Resistant to changes seen all over the rest of Boston, it still had aromas peculiar to the old country's style of Italian cooking. For centuries, it had been an enclave for immigrants, from the days of silversmith Paul Revere when a mix of wealthy and laboring classes shared the small area, to the influx of Irish and Eastern European Jews. The latest and most lasting population was first-, second-, and third-generation Italians, and when Bostonians think of the North End now, they think of a predominantly Italian community.

Luckily, he'd made reservations for a back room at Luca's. It was packed as usual. This was a watering hole for a select group of the town's political and business movers and shakers. Tom saw the mayor of Boston and the Massachusetts Speaker of the House huddled in conspiratorial conversation in one corner. In another cul-de-sac he saw the president of Commonwealth Bank laughing at some remark by a new prominence in the business community, the owner of a recently opened casino. He hoped there were no pharmaceutical executives eating dinner there if conversation got loud from his board. He sat between Eileen Givens, a journalist, and Yolanda Jefferson, one of the community representatives.

"Happy with your board?" Eileen asked.

"Delighted. What a talented group!"

"I have a suggestion for you," Yolanda said. "In order to snag public interest in our mission, use examples of actual people who've suffered from the pharmaceutical industry's questionable behaviors to get your points across.

People latch onto stories with a human face. That makes it easier for them to grasp underlying issues."

"I agree completely," said Eileen. "After twenty-five years in journalism, experience tells me all lead columns begin with a human-interest story."

"So, how do we find particular cases that will illustrate our issues?" Tom asked.

"Social media," Yolanda said. "Get on it early and often. And get our website active. Ask people to tell us their complaints about problems with access and price and all the other things we talked about." Tom caught the words "our website" and recognized that at least this board member already identified with PharmaTruth. "I'll bet you'll get tons of responses. Sort them out, get staff to interview people and go from there."

"The other thing is that you and board members need to get out and talk to groups," Eileen said. "Church groups, advocacy groups, veterans, AARP local clubs, Kiwanis, Chamber of Commerce, anyone who might have a stake in this, which means everyone, really. Seek out key media people to give you newspaper and television coverage."

"How do we coordinate this?" Tom asked, in his best Socratic method.

"A public relations director," Eileen said. "And a techie who maintains a website that's attractive and user-friendly, avoiding barriers between us and people using it. Answers calls. A sure path to failure is to ask for help and then make it hard for callers to get through to key people. It's like being on call as a doctor. You're familiar with that, right? You gotta take calls and answer their questions. There'll be some crank calls, of course, but they can be handled. It's a lot of work and it's time-intense, but it'll pay off."

Tom dictated these ideas into his cellphone as he left Luca's. Then he remembered he'd planned to tell the board about hiring Burseik. *Completely forgot that. Damn.* But his mind was dwelling on Cynthia and the dinner with her.

***

Tom pulled open the Red Fez's heavy oak door, pushed a maroon drape back and was led to a booth. He fidgeted with the menu without reading it and glanced around, recalling meals he'd eaten here while a surgical resident at Boston Medical Center. Not much had changed, a reassuring sign in a city that was continually being altered by rampant new construction, high-rise condo complexes, horrendous traffic, and a host of impatient people, slaves to their technology.

Cynthia strode in, her tall slender frame silhouetted and her dark hair reflecting lights in the entryway. Tom had always loved her hooded brown eyes and the contours of her cheeks and bow-like mouth. She would never be mistaken for a fashion model, not beautiful that way, but there was an aura about her that never failed to turn heads. She'd worn Tom's requested Asian-print scarf and it complemented her dark blue silk dress.

Tom stood to greet her, they hugged, tentatively at first, then warmly and for a long time. They parted, still touching and looked at each other at arm's length, trying to understand their feelings. Both brushed tears away as they sat down in the booth.

"Well, aren't we the sappy ones?" Cynthia said.

"I knew this would happen. Couple of sentimental slobs," Tom agreed.

"I guess we should forgive ourselves. We have a colorful past," Cynthia laughed. "So, have you seen Akira or Dr. Goodfellow or Alicia?"

"I saw Akira briefly when we started PharmaTruth, but I've been so busy trying to get it off the ground that I've neglected my old friends. By the way, I brought you a brochure that describes what we're trying to do."

"I suppose you expect me to contribute money," she said, grinning.

"Hell yes, I expect at least a million from you. A rich dean of nursing. You can write a check or put it on your credit card."

"Forgot both and I only have enough cash for this dinner," she responded in kind. "By the way, this dinner is on me. I called this meeting so it's my treat. No, don't object, it's decided.

"Shall we order? I'm famished. Skipped lunch."

Her hands shook as she perused the menu. Tom saw that he was not the only one nervous.

"Mind if I have a drink? Are you still forbidden?" Cynthia asked.

"I'm careful about alcohol but I guess a glass of wine can't hurt."

They ordered and when food came, they ate like they were back on call, exchanging glances between filling their mouths, feeling anxious about where conversation might lead. They laid their utensils down in unison as the race to the end of feeding ended.

"What terrific food," Cynthia said. "Good choice. I remember coming here often but wasn't sure it was still here."

"Always loved this place. I don't recognize the woman who seated me, but I bet they have the same chef."

Safe talk so far.

"Well. I guess I should begin," Cynthia said. "First off, I'm sorry I called everything off back then. Seems like a long time ago. I was scared even though I didn't really believe you would assault me again, either physically or verbally. I knew medication had made a difference in your symptoms. But our whole relationship was like a patient with multiple systems failure, so many things going wrong at once. You understand what I'm saying?"

"It did seem hopeless at times," Tom said. "We both kept swimming while we were in the midst of it, but once we reached an island and could breathe again, it looked different in our exhaustion. To me, too. It felt like we needed too much help to keep our love alive."

"As I told you on the phone, time has given me perspective," Cynthia said. "I look back and feel like I was a selfish coward. This self-loathing has only gotten worse the further away from our break-up." Tears formed as she took another sip of wine.

"Just so you know," Tom said, "*Self*-loathing aside, I don't loathe you, and I'm not angry with you. I've gained perspective too and have thought about this often. I'm still very fond of you. My first real love. A ton of love songs about that."

"Well, I don't know how to say this. I guess I'd like for us to find out if there's anything left from those days. Could you consider giving it another chance?"

Tom felt dizzy as he considered this. In his heart, he'd hoped someday they might get back together.

"How would we go about it?" he asked in honest confusion.

"Gradually. I think meeting for dinner occasionally, maybe going to a concert or a game. Nothing requiring much, other than getting acquainted again. Then see how it goes. I'm as apprehensive as you seem to be, so we're starting out at the same place."

"You're right. Frankly, I'm wary about this. But I'm willing to meet occasionally and, as you say, see how things go."

Cynthia slumped a little in her chair sensing that Tom's enthusiasm seemed tepid.

"I'm wary too," she said. "But I'm apparently more hopeful than you are. If you don't want to do this, I understand."

"As I said, I'm willing to give it a try," Tom said hurriedly, trying to convey more interest than his response had so far. "But you know this could be painful and even dangerous for us. Painful because we'll revisit old demons and dangerous because we could have another bad ending." He recalled an old poem about shirking pain and losing happiness as well.

"The ball is in your court. Call me when you've decided," she said evenly as she reached for the check and nodded to the waitress.

"Like to meet in Worcester next time so you don't have to drive into Boston?" Tom asked, trying to display his enthusiasm for this desirable venture.

"That would be nice, though I kinda like coming back into Boston. Brings back pleasant memories."

Cynthia paid the bill, and they left together. She reached her car and said, "Wanna ride?"

"Sure. Can you drop me off at my place on Beacon Hill?" Tom said.

"Glad to. Hop in."

Cynthia eased her car into traffic and asked for directions.

"Like living on Beacon Hill?"

"It's great. My apartment was recently renovated, spacious for this area, and I'm in easy walking distance from my office. And if I need medical attention there's the World's Greatest Hospital down the hill."

"You don't need any medical attention, do you?" she asked apprehensively.

"No, I'm fine," Tom laughed. "My arm is the same, always will be, and the rest of my body's in pretty good shape. Oh, here's the building. Thanks for the lift." He leaned over and planted a kiss on her lips, surprising them both. "Still a good kisser, I see," he said.

"Same for you. Thanks for meeting me. See you next time." Cynthia said.

"Thanks for dinner and for reaching out. I'm very glad you did. I'll call soon. I've enjoyed tonight. See you later."

Tom watched as she drove off, filled with ambivalence—warmth, fear, hope.

Chapter 6

As he emerged from Cynthia's car, Tom turned to unlock his door and caught the aroma of cigarette smoke. He quickly scanned entryways in both directions and noticed the glow of a cigarette in one. A shudder of fear went through him, recalling the security warnings raised by Amitav Kumar. Was he being watched? Or was this only someone having a smoke outside of their condo?

He opened his door, turned on a light and bolted the door behind him. His eyes danced around the room to detect any changes since he was last home. Nothing seemed different as he passed through each room. The pounding in his head subsided as he poured himself a glass of sherry and checked his messages, most unimportant. Except for one.

"Tom, sorry I missed you. I wanted to apologize for my abrupt departure the other night. I was so freaked about being late for the babysitter that I was very inconsiderate. Hope you got home okay. When you have a chance, please give me a call."

This took Tom by surprise, and he felt a bit disoriented, having just left Cynthia. *What could she be calling about?* He glanced at his watch – 10:45 p.m. Still early evening in La Jolla. He dialed Katharine's number. She picked up right away.

"Hi. Tom here. Just got in and got your message. How're you doing?"

"Oh, Tom, thanks for calling. Can you hold on a sec? I need to go into another room to talk. The kids are jumping around, getting ready for bed."

"I can call back if that would be easier."

"Could you? 'Bout a half hour?"

He visualized her inviting face and imagined he could smell her hair. The next half hour crept by as he waited to call.

"Tom? Thanks for calling back."

"Good to hear your voice. How's it going?" he said, wondering what this was about.

"Pretty well. In my rush to get home the other night I didn't thank you properly for making the trip out to see me. The other thing is, talking with you allowed me to tap into many issues I've run away from. I'd like to continue that conversation."

"I enjoyed being with you, sharing our feelings. I think it was good for both of us. But I agree with you. A lot was left unsaid."

"Yeah, so true. I thought we only began to get into some, well, important and pretty distressing personal things."

Tom hesitated. Cautious about this new terrain, his curiosity impelled him to respond.

"I felt that too," he said. "But I'm wondering if this is better to do in person rather than by phone," Tom recognized his avoidance behavior clicking in.

"Are you coming back to the West Coast anytime?" Katharine said with an uptick in her voice.

"No plans to, but I can arrange to come out."

"Well, let me tell you what's on my mind. I wanted to pursue something that has haunted me since I was notified of Danny's death." Katharine shifted the phone from one ear to the other as she drew in a deep breath. "You were one of the last persons to see Danny alive. You know where and how it happened. As I told you, his death is so, I don't know, abstract and unreal to me. It's never seemed real. I know that sounds odd, but maybe it's partly because I'm a scientist, partly a spiritual thing." She stopped. "Am I making any sense? "It's just that I never saw his body, only the container of his remains. Sounds awful to say such a thing, but it's hard to believe he died when I don't have any real proof. I don't even know for sure where it happened. Can you understand this?"

"Yes. I've seen a lot of death, personally and as a doctor. And you're right, it's hard to get your mind around losing a loved one if you're not there when it happens." He recalled his disbelief when his mother told him his father had died. "What do you think would help make it real, less abstract for you, make it possible to accept the fact of Danny's death?"

"Talking to you helped, how you bore witness to his death. I think another way might be visiting where it happened."

"I can tell you that I was talking to Danny minutes before he died. I saw the results of the explosion. I'm one hundred percent sure Danny was killed in that explosion. I saw the hospital room after the bomb detonated." Tom couldn't tell her he'd seen Danny's shattered body along with the nurses on the floor of the operating suite. "Is that helpful for me to tell you that?"

"It is. I believe you and appreciate your being able to tell me." She unconsciously slipped her hand over her heart. "That helps a lot."

"About seeing where it happened," Tom continued. "That's hard. The Middle East is a tangled web of politics, violence, corruption and unpredictability. I'm not sure a private citizen could go to the site where it actually occurred. The whole place is a war zone. Added to that, finding exactly where would be difficult, because our unit moved from place to place."

As Tom thought about this, his Commanding Officer, Colonel Benjamin Higgins came to mind. He wondered where he was now.

"Finding where we were would require military assistance using historical records of that engagement, probably geographical coordinates, and I don't know what else. My instincts tell me it's a long shot."

"I know going there is unrealistic. But even being able to spot a place on the map would help."

"I'll try to locate our Commanding Officer and see if he could help. Finding Colonel Higgins shouldn't be hard. The military keeps good records of their personnel. Let me pursue that. I'll call you in a few days."

"Tom, you're wonderful, you're a love. Let me know what you find out. Just talking to you has been so helpful. Thanks."

After Tom hung up, the word "love" lingered in his mind. He visualized Katharine's long dark hair, her brown eyes, her slim body. He felt a warm rush. Then a different feeling, confusion, overtook him. The recollection of his wonderful reunion with Cynthia crowded in and muddled his thoughts. *Can I be in love with two women at the same time?*

The next day, after a few calls, he tracked down Colonel Higgins. He was retired and living in Coronado, California. Right outside of San Diego! He called him and a woman answered.

"Hello, my name is Dr. Tom Barrett and I'm looking for Colonel Higgins. He was my CO when we were in Iraq. Is this the correct number?"

"Yes, this is his wife. What did you say your name was? Ben is upstairs in his study."

A few minutes later Higgins' familiar voice was booming through the phone.

"Tom, how are you? Where are you?"

"I'm fine. I'm calling from Boston. So good to hear your voice. You're retired?"

"Yes, and glad of it. What're you doing?"

Tom told him about PharmaTruth briefly and then told him his reason for calling.

"Colonel, I promised Danny Mott that if anything happened to him, I'd reach out to his wife. I've met with her a couple of times and recently talked with her by phone. She lives in La Jolla, incidentally."

"That was good of you Tom. I still remember that horrific day. How is she coping? They had a couple of kids, right?"

"Yes. She's doing reasonably well, but like many war widows she has trouble believing her husband is really dead. She has recurrent dreams of his coming home. I think I've convinced her about the reality of his death, but she thinks knowing the exact location of his death would help. Is there any way to pin that down?"

"I think I have the location of our unit in my files. Let me poke around."

"You're in Coronado and she's in La Jolla," Tom said as he mulled over what to do. "Maybe the three of us could get together and you could talk to her in person. I think that would make it even more real for her. It also would be great for me to see you again."

"I could do that. Let me call you when I've had some time to locate the files, okay? Listen, really good to hear from you. I'll call you soon."

Higgins had always been a scrupulous officer. On this matter, he was true to his habit and called a day later.

"Tom, I've found those files. I can pinpoint our exact location at that time from the coordinates. What I thought I'd do is generate a map, highlight the spot and get this to Katharine. What do you think of that idea?"

"I think it's the right thing to do, Colonel." He gave Katharine's phone number, email and address to him, then paused, wrestling with the consideration of flying back to San Diego to be with her when Higgins presented the map. "What's your plan on giving this to her?"

"I could call her and meet with her and give it to her in person. Does that seem okay?"

"I think that would be fine. Would you like me to join you?"

"You're welcome to do that. But don't feel it's necessary for you to fly back out here for this. But it's completely up to you."

"Thank you, Colonel. Above and beyond, as they say."

Chapter 7

Rose Robbins crashed down hard on her wood deck stairs. She was lugging a potted philodendron plant from her family room over the deck when she tripped over a couple of forgotten pots she'd been planting herbs in earlier. The lush plant went flying, settling on the lawn near where Rose landed, her left leg twisted at a gruesome angle. Pain shot up through her hip, so extreme that she passed out. When she awoke, the pain was still excruciating but she was able to grope for her phone to dial 911. The dispatcher, after determining her whereabouts, sent an ambulance to transport her to Lakeville Community Hospital.

"You have a broken hip bone in what's called the femoral neck," the orthopedist said with no preliminary comforting words after he'd read the x-rays. "It's pretty bad, displaced and angulated. You need surgery. As soon as we get you cleared, and we get an operating room ready we'll put you back together. I need you to sign permissions for anesthesia and surgery. Do you have a relative we can call for you?"

Still bewildered by what had happened and drowsy from painkillers, she stared at the yellow privacy curtains encircling her, then the ceiling tiles. Medical paraphernalia hung all over the walls, a blinking computer screen stared at her, and this impersonal stranger in a blue scrub suit whose name tag she couldn't read was looking down on her.

"My daughter's name is Dina Robbins. She lives in Needham. Please call her. Don't alarm her, tell her I'm doing fine but would like her to come here. Thank you for all you've done." The doctor seemed to dissolve in a hazy cloud.

Nurses threw warming blankets over Rose once she was in the operating room. People were busy with all manner of chores Rose couldn't understand. Another stranger in blue scrubs hovered over her and introduced herself as Carolyn, nurse anesthetist. She asked questions about her past experiences with anesthesia, drug and latex allergies, medications she took, and on and on. Rose took a deep breath, answered as best she could and then lapsed into an anesthetic funk. Later, when she opened her eyes, she was in a different room. A new contingent of scrubs-clad personnel was bustling around.

"Oh, you're awake," a nurse said in a cheerful voice. "Welcome to our recovery room. I'm Amy, and I'll be taking care of you while you're here. Your doctor will be in to see you shortly. Anything I can do for you right now?"

Rose's eyes flickered, trying to focus, her brain doing its best to get oriented. She felt no pain but had a sense of floating in a large vat of jelly. She finally was able to answer, "No, I don't need anything right now, thanks." The nurse adjusted her blankets, injected something into her IV tubing and disappeared. Rose drifted back into a fog. When she awoke, she looked into her daughter's face.

"Mom? Can you hear me?" Dina asked.

"Oh sweetie, thank goodness you're here. I'm so confused. Everything happened so suddenly. I'm sorry to cause all this trouble."

"Mom, you didn't fall down on purpose."

"I forgot about the herb pots...couldn't see over the plant...so stupid...I'm sorry."

"Stop apologizing. I'm so happy to see you in such good shape. When they called and told me what happened, I was terrified. You really had a terrible break in your hip bone. The doctor showed me the x-ray, but he was able to fix it. So, don't worry. I'm here and can stay as long as you need me."

"Can they spare you at the nursing school? What about Debbie?"

"Of course. No classes for several days. Besides, you're more important than my classes. And you know Debbie's not a little girl anymore; you were at her seventeenth birthday, remember? She can take care of herself."

Rose went back to sleep and Dina slipped away to talk with Amy.

"Just so you know, I'm a nurse but I promise not to interfere," Dina smiled and winked. "I hope you'll keep me informed not only as her daughter but as a fellow professional who needs to know everything. Okay?"

"Sure. Want to get on some scrubs and help out?" Amy laughed.

"Nope, I'm gonna try to behave myself," Dina said.

Mom, you're the best person in the world, and I'll make sure you get the best care, Dina thought.

While Rose slept, Dina called the school, told them where she was and why, that she'd be back next week. She figured Rose would begin light physical therapy by then and wouldn't need her constant presence. For now, she'd sleep in Rose's room on a fold-out chair. First, though, she called her daughter.

"Debbie? Grandma took a spill and broke her hip. She's in Lakeville Hospital, they operated, and I'm with her. Looks like I'll be here a few days. You okay? There's plenty of food there and if you don't see what you'd like, just eat out and I'll reimburse you."

"I'm okay, but poor Grandma. Broke her leg? Jeez, how awful. What's gonna happen?"

"I haven't spoken to her doctor yet, but can you please call Rabbi Cohen to let him know?"

"Sure. Should I call Dad?"

"Are you kidding? Why should he care now after all these years of total neglect?" Divorced right after Dina got pregnant with Debbie, he'd simply deserted them. He had very limited contact, although Debbie saw him occasionally, and she still wanted a relationship with him. Probably thought this would be an opportunity to spend some time together. He seemed always to need an "event" to see her.

"Should I come visit her?"

"Yes, but not right now. She's a little confused and needs to rest and get better. When she's more herself, you should come see her."

***

Rose woke up during the third postoperative night complaining of being hot. A nurse took her temperature. She had fever of 101 degrees.

"Will you talk to the doctor?" Dina asked. *Not a good sign.*

"He'll be around in a couple of hours to see her on morning rounds."

"Can the resident have a look at her now?"

"I could call him, but he'll probably wait until rounds to see her."

"Dina, sweetie, don't bother the doctor. He needs his sleep," Rose said, overhearing this conversation. Rose never wanted to inconvenience anyone.

"A postop fever is not to be ignored," Dina said, breaking out of her preferred role as daughter and involuntarily assuming a nurse's perspective. She looked at the nurse and sternly said, "I'd appreciate it if you called the resident."

"Okay, I'll call him," the nurse said as she walked away.

She's probably silently swearing at me and thinks I'm a hovering daughter. I couldn't care less. Maybe this one doesn't know I'm a nurse. But even if I weren't, she should be doing her job without my insistence. What do ordinary patients do when they don't have a health professional overseeing their hospital care? Nurses are supposed to be patient advocates. Okay, stop kvetching. But still...

A sleepy resident came in, glanced at Dina, mumbled a hello. He greeted Rose and asked her to sit up a little so he could listen to her back.

"Her lungs are clear. She's a little warm. Let's see what her temp is now."

Dina saw the temperature was up to 103.

"Mmm, gone up a couple of degrees. Rose, do you have any pain where you were operated?" the resident asked.

"Well, it's hard to tell with all these pain pills I've had. But it does feel a little sore."

The resident pulled back the covers, palpated over the surgical site. Rose winced. "Yes, that hurts when you do that."

He unwrapped the bandages to look at the wound and saw what all surgeons fear: angry red flesh over the surgical site with a few beads of pus oozing from the surgical wound. Now he was concerned.

"Get me culture swabs and blood culture tubes," he told the nurse. "And give her 1000 milligrams of acetaminophen."

The resident moved quickly to do what Dina knew had to be done. As soon as blood cultures and wound swabs were taken, intravenous antibiotics were flowing. Dina prayed that the infection was not MRSA – methicillin-resistant staphylococcus aureus – a dreaded organism that was the bane of surgeons.

Dina paced in Rose's room, looking out the window, stomach churning, heart racing. Rose's temperature had stubbornly stayed at 103 and she was uncomfortable most of the next day.

"We're taking new blood cultures and moving your mother to the Intensive Care Unit," the surgical resident told Dina late in the afternoon. "I'm sorry you won't be able to sleep there, but we've prepared a sleeping room for you across the hall." Dina was treated with great deference since she'd been right about getting the resident out of bed to care for her mother. Malpractice suits were feared in hospitals almost as much as MRSA.

By day five, Rose's temperature continued to hover around 103. She was more disoriented, waking during the night with sweats and hallucinations.

"MRSA has grown out of her last blood cultures," the resident said. "We're starting a different antibiotic." He put his hand on Dina's arm. "I must be honest. This is not good news." He looked at Dina. She leaned against him, losing her composure and crying softly. She could no longer watch staff ministering to her mother.

After the resident led her to her sleeping room, she called Debbie but couldn't let her know how scared she was. She didn't want to alarm her by asking her to come right away.

"Rabbi Cohen? This is Dina Robbins. I know you stopped by a couple of days ago, but Mom has gotten so much worse. She's got a resistant bug in her bloodstream, and she looks awful. Up 'til now I thought she would beat this, she's always been so healthy, but now… I'm scared, Rabbi. She could die," she sobbed. "Could you come, please?"

He came quickly, hearing the urgency and distress in Dina's voice. Although glad he could offer comfort, nothing he could say made this better.

Was her mother going to die? Why wasn't the antibiotic working?

As they sat together, she told Rabbi Cohen that she knew MRSA was a stubborn infection. "But it isn't always fatal, you know." She then took refuge in her nursing knowledge. "In fact, mortality rate is low in studies on whole populations, but considerably higher in older people," she said. "But Mom is in her early 70's and has always been in good health, so I'm sure she's not as vulnerable as most older people." She tried to keep up her hopes.

Rabbi Cohen stayed with Dina for over two hours. When Rose was sleeping comfortably, he left, and Dina went to the on-call room to rest. Out of the din of the intensive care unit, her mind turned to her interests since becoming a nurse. A lecturer in pharmacology, she'd found the study of drugs and their therapeutic applications, side-effects and interactions to be a consuming passion. She could get lost in an intricate web of chemical compounds and how they affect cells and organs. The irony of her own mother being the terrain on which a war between a fierce bacterial invader and a pharmacological agent was taking place was not lost on her. She prayed to a god she doubted existed to spare her mother.

The next morning the doctors told Dina they were changing antibiotics again to one that appeared more promising in the sensitivity studies, but not to hold out false hopes. She knew this new antibiotic had a slightly better record for MRSA and was somewhat encouraged. The next twenty-four hours would be critical.

***

"Your mother's fever is not coming down," said Dr. Aiken, director of the intensive care unit. "Despite the sensitivity studies the infection is not responding to the new antibiotic. As you know, MRSA is a stubborn bug. And for reasons we don't understand, her renal function is going downhill. Does she have a history of kidney disease?"

"She had surgery as a child for urinary tract reflux and double collecting systems, but has had no trouble since, that

I know of," Dina said. "Wait, now that I think back, she might have had urinary tract infections. When I was young, she used to take pills, said they were for 'water problems.' Never thought much about it. Maybe what she meant was kidney or bladder problems, maybe infections."

"Well, her blood urea nitrogen is sky-high and her other kidney function tests are off," Dr. Aiken said. "I don't think the antibiotics are responsible for that. She may have had undiagnosed kidney disease for some time and this illness is unmasking it. We'll consult our nephrologist to advise us."

Dina went to Rose's ICU cubicle, trying to be quiet, but her mother was awake.

"Hello dear, come in. I'm not feeling so good today," Rose said.

Dina took her hand. "Anything you need?"

"Only to get out of here. Have you been over to my house? My plants need water, I'm sure," she said. "How are you doing? You've been here a lot. Hope they don't fire you for not coming to work! And how's Debbie?"

"No chance of getting fired. And Debbie's coming to see you soon. I told her to wait until you were better. Maybe she can come tonight."

"I'd love to see her. She still going out with that nice boy?"

"To be honest Mom, I'm not sure. She doesn't talk much about her boyfriends to her old-fashioned mother."

A knock on the door frame got the attention of Dina and Rose.

"Excuse me, I'm Dr. Kaminsky from the Nephrology Service. I was asked to see Rose Robbins. Am I in the right place?"

"Yes, I'm her daughter and this is Rose," Dina said, stepping away from the bed. "May I stay while you talk to Mom?"

"Sure, that would be ideal."

He proceeded to take a long, detailed history, examined Rose, and told her he'd be back later when he'd had a chance to look at her records in more detail. Dina followed him hoping to find out what he thought.

"As you know her renal function studies are quite abnormal. I need radiology to help, so we'll get appropriate studies and then I may be able to tell you more," Dr. Kaminsky said.

"Thanks so much. I'll be here and would like to be kept informed. I'm a nurse-pharmacologist and her daughter, so I hope you won't hold back sharing information."

"Not at all. You'll be kept fully informed."

Over the next two days Rose underwent several radiological exams. The results, however, were not encouraging.

"She's lost a lot of renal tissue, and the function is not good. If she were younger and not on IV antibiotics, she might be a candidate for a kidney transplant, but under her circumstances we can't even offer dialysis until the infection is cleared up," Dr. Kaminsky said. "How long her kidneys will hold up while she's getting over her sepsis is hard to predict. So, we'll just have to take it a day at a time."

Dina took a deep breath and sighed. *How long would it have been until we found out about her kidney disease had she not broken her hip,* she wondered. *How long until the buildup of urea and other toxins in the blood interfere with everything else?*

That question was answered that night. Her mental state deteriorated, and the heart monitor showed signs of arrhythmias. The doctors anxiously drew blood to determine her potassium levels.

"Code Blue Room 402!" the overhead speaker blared. A half dozen staff rushed into Rose's room and saw her convulsing wildly. They hurried to her side, pushing anticonvulsant meds into her IV line. Her arrhythmia got worse. Dina leaped out of bed and rushed across the hall when she heard the code called. She stood powerlessly at the door to Rose's room, pressing her fingers against her temples as she watched Rose in her final throes. The straight line on the heart monitor was devastating to watch.

She cried, with sobs rising from deep within her. *What else could I have been done? How do these things happen? An accidental fall, good surgical outcome, then infection triggering a sequence of horrid biological events, uncovering unforeseen and hidden vulnerabilities of the flesh.*

Dina grieved. *I thought Mom was a healthy 72- year-old woman. How could she be gone?*

Chapter 8

The petroleum scent of recently laid carpeting still hung in the air. Computers and phone banks were pristine in PharmaTruth's new quarters. In his office, Tom turned on his computer and scrutinized PharmaTruth's Home Page.

Okay, our website is live. Let's see some activity.

PharmaTruth
Our Mission: Shine a Light on Questionable
Practices of Pharmaceutical Companies.

**This free website was created for information
exchanges between our staff and people who
have had difficulty obtaining drugs because:**
Drugs are priced out of your reach.
Your insurance is insufficient for payment.

This website is for people who are:
Confused and frustrated by advertisements about
drugs.
Health care providers who object to misleading
information about drug research.

Health care providers fed up with pharmaceutical companies trying to manipulate their prescribing practices.
Addicted to opiates because a doctor over-prescribed OxyContin or Oxycodone

**Use this website for complaints about Pharma lawyers negotiating modest settlements for claims of adverse drug events.
Call 617-555-0000 to talk with one of our representatives.
www.PharmaTruth.org**

"Any media coverage yet?" Dolores asked, standing in the doorway.

"Those two interviews with TV stations are scheduled for this week, and Eileen placed ads in local newspapers and in three national news services," Tom said. "She's also written two Op-Ed articles for four major newspapers. If we're flooded with responses, we'll have to find more volunteers to field calls. That would be an embarrassment of riches, wouldn't it?"

Looking out over the ten cubicles in the office, Tom watched Emily, one of the volunteers, taking a call. When she hung up, she handed him a message.

"Thanks," he said, and read, "My name is Dr. Norman Wise. I'm a practicing internist in Boston. I saw your website. I'd like to talk to someone confidentially and in person."

"He left this telephone number and email address," Emily said. "He seemed a little hesitant when I first answered. He wanted to know who I was and when I told him I was a volunteer, he said he'd wanted to talk with someone in charge. I gave him your name and told him that I'd pass his message on to you."

"I'll give him a call. Thanks Emily."

Tom was intrigued. *What's behind the call? Is it an opening salvo in a sure- to-come battle with big Pharma? But a practicing internist wouldn't be part of a pharmaceutical company, would he? Well, he could be. I'll have the researcher check out his authenticity – at least we'll know that much. Should I call him right away or wait a day or two? He said he wanted to talk, when I know he's who he says he is, I'll just do it.*

Later, Tom left a message with Dr. Wise's receptionist and got busy with other things. A return phone call came in quickly.

"This is Dr. Tom Barrett. You wanted to speak to me?"

"Yes, thanks for getting back to me," Dr. Wise said. After a couple of beats, he said, "Um, would it be possible for us to meet?"

"Yes, of course. Can you tell me why?"

"Not on the phone. Could you meet me at the George Washington statue in Boston Garden? We can find a place to talk from there."

Tom's stomach tightened, his eye twitched. *Get a grip, he told himself. A meeting like that is in broad daylight. You're not going to be abducted again, not in Boston Garden.*

"Okay, when would you like to do this?"

"I have no office hours tomorrow. Could we meet at noon? Is that at all possible?"

"Tomorrow noon is fine," Tom said. Then, "How will I know you?"

"I'll be wearing a black leather jacket and an Irish cap. I'm middle-aged, have a white beard, about 5-10, white."

Tom described himself to Dr. Wise and hung up.

He was apprehensive. He didn't like clandestine meetings, but he was curious. An image of his old pal and fellow patient at Zylinski, George Logan, popped into his mind: Black, small- town Alabamian, head neatly shaven, wire-rim glasses. Big guy. *Must be around 33 or 34 by now, Tom mused. Soft-spoken but when he spoke people listened. Of course, just the guy I need, he thought. He told me to call if I ever needed him. I think I need him now.*

Tom scrolled through his phone directory. He found the number of the detective agency George had given him the last time they were at a follow-up appointment at Zylinski when he had given George a rough idea of PharmaTruth.

When George answered after the first ring, Tom said, "George, good to hear your voice. What's happenin' man?"

"Are you talking Black English to me?" George teased. "Not a good imitation of our speech, and coming from you, an elite, honkey doctor, it just doesn't work."

"I tried," Tom said, smiling at the familiar banter with George. "So, still enjoying the detective business?"

"It's a living, but it's boring. Following unfaithful husbands around to catch them being naughty isn't my idea of private investigation. But it pays the bills."

"How would you like to work for my outfit?" Tom's mouth jumped ahead of his mental processing. "I think I need you for a lot of things, including protecting my sorry ass. You could start tomorrow. Salary negotiable."

"What? You kidding me?"

"Not at all. I have a meeting tomorrow in Boston Garden at noon with 'a mysterious stranger.'" Tom chuckled as he uttered the pulp mystery fiction cliché. "Know almost nothing about him and frankly, I'm nervous. While you're thinking about my offer, could you find time to hang around George Washington's statue in the Garden and watch this meeting go down?"

"I could do that. Lunch hour, you know?" He laughed, and then picked up on Tom's proposition. "Can we get together and talk more about your offer? I'm interested."

"Maybe after I talk with this guy in Boston Garden you could come to my office. I can fill you in on what we're doing with PharmaTruth."

"Okay, I'll stay inconspicuous, and then I'll trail you to your office."

"Always the pro, George. See you." Tom felt more relaxed already.

***

Doctor Wise stood squarely in front of Washington's statue. He was easy to spot. His face was long, nose canted to one side, and his white beard was close-cropped. One could tell he was a fastidious man. Looking left and right, Tom saw another man, hidden by the newspaper he was reading, sitting on a bench nearby. He hoped it was George. Tom moved towards the doctor with an outstretched hand.

"I'm Tom Barrett. You must be Dr. Wise."

"Right. Good to meet you," he said, glancing around in several directions. "I think we can sit over there," he said, motioning toward a park bench.

"I'm sure you're wondering what this is about," Wise said. "Well, I guess it's my way of assuaging guilt for what I've done in cahoots with a drug company. It's been a gradual slide into the betrayal of my medical oath." He sighed. "So, here's my story.

"I have a thriving private cardiology practice. About three years ago, a drug rep who'd been generous in supplying me with some quite expensive sample drugs that I provide for patients with low income, asked if I'd be interested in speaking to a small select group of doctors over dinner at an upscale restaurant in downtown Boston. A nice honorarium was to be provided. Flattered, I accepted his offer. This led to more and more speaking gigs."

"Did he pay you for these talks?"

"No, he didn't pay me directly. The honorarium he mentioned came from attendees who paid to come. But, out of a sense of obligation for arranging these speaking opportunities, I, of course, prescribed drugs made by his company to the exclusion of competitor's drugs and told patients that generic drugs weren't as good, and even told some they weren't safe."

"So, you can't say you were overtly bribed in any way?"

"Not directly."

Dr. Wise stared off into the Boston sky looking sad, struggling with words. "The drug rep asked me to do, um, other things. He paid me for giving my advice about the effectiveness of 'marketing campaigns.' He also paid me to listen to and evaluate other sales reps delivering their sales pitches." Wise took off his cap and smoothed his hair, his lower lip quivering. "Then he asked me to participate in 'studies' that paid me for each patient I'd put on a particular drug. Turns out these were not 'studies' at all, but gimmicks to increase the number of prescriptions I'd write. I'd been misled, taken for the fool I was."

"This probably took a fair amount of time," Tom said, trying to be sympathetic to a guy obviously drowning in guilt.

"It grew to about a quarter of my time and income. Easy money. No risk involved. No after-hours calls. And, as I said, built up support for..." Wise stood up, turned to face Tom.

"I'm not done," Wise said in almost a whisper. "The drug rep sent company-employed doctors and pharmacologists to my office, ostensibly to educate me about their newest drugs, to prepare me to give more lectures. They even supplied me with power-point presentations with impressive, colorful graphs. Because they were peers, not drug salespeople, I believed what they told me. With authority, these 'fellow professionals' described unapproved off-brand uses of these drugs. I began prescribing them for those purposes and telling colleagues to do the same."

"This piled up on your conscience, made you ashamed," Tom said, trying to be supportive.

Dr. Wise nodded.

"A lot like doing unnecessary surgery, the area I'm most familiar with." Tom said, shifting in his seat and pulling his left arm up across his lap.

"I'm glad you contacted me," Tom said. "Not sure how to use this, but I'd like to stay in touch. As we pull together evidence about unethical activities like those you've described, someday we'll find a way to have legislative hearings to expose them. But we need to proceed deliberately, not jump the gun and have it back-fire."

"If it comes to those hearings, I'm willing to testify," Dr. Wise said firmly. "I must be careful, though, not to show I'm no longer their stooge. I'll have to continue to cooperate with their schemes to avoid suspicion. No telling what they might do to damage my professional reputation."

"I'd also be careful about your personal safety. Not to alarm you, but I was the victim of substantial harm by a drug company," Tom said looking at his limp arm.

Dr. Wise glanced at Tom's arm and went pale.

Tom gave him his secure phone number and email so he could communicate without fear of discovery. Dr. Wise walked away toward Commonwealth Avenue. Tom looked around for George, found him, elbows on the stone bridge spanning a channel connecting two ponds, watching the fish. Casually, George looked around and nodded, letting Tom know he'd be behind him.

Back at Mt. Vernon Street, Tom showed the headquarters to George. "He didn't look very threatening." George laughed.

"Turns out he's been manipulated by a drug house, and he's spilled his guts to me. He feels guilty and wants to atone."

Tom gave George a brochure, grabbed some coffee and bagels for them and ushered him into his office, closing the door quietly.

"Nice place," George said. "I'm impressed. Who would've thought you'd be running a big-time organization when we hovered over you in that deep coma? We all thought you were a goner. But look at you now!"

"Well, if it hadn't been for you and Matt, I'd be a goner as you so delicately put it. I'll never forget what you did. It's not hard for me to offer you a job heading up our Security Unit. You'll have a blank slate because I don't know exactly how we'll use a Security Unit. But I know you'll figure it out."

"Is there a salary?" George grinned.

"Does $100,000 annual sound okay to you as a start?"

"Actually, $125,000 sounds better. Can you do that? I'm still paying off bills from my parents' last days," George said.

"Agreed. As I think about this, my friend Amitav Kumar, who runs an industry watchdog corporation in San Francisco, comes to mind. He has tight security in his organization. You could call him and get information as to how he set his unit up, maybe talk to someone there. We need similar protection at PharmaTruth for the same reasons. You'll need a budget with flexibility for the Security Unit. Equipment. Perhaps additional staff. I admit I'm paranoid. The other night at my condo I smelled cigarette smoke as I got out of my cab and thought I saw a glow down the street. Probably nothing, but it scared me.

"I'll work out a proposal and let you dissect it, expand it if need be. I want the whole place protected.

"Now let's find an office for you, introduce you to Dolores, who runs my life here. You'll like her, but be careful, she's dangerous," Tom said with a smile.

Chapter 9

"Tom. Akira calling. Have time to talk?"

"Akira! Of course, I can talk to you. Anytime."

"Sorry I haven't called sooner but, you know, the Institute keeps making demands. I wanted to know how your new venture is going. Also wanted to tell you about news on one of your friends.

"Progress is moving forward nicely. Let's get together; I'll fill you in on what we're doing." *Wonder which friend Akira was referring to. Could it be Akira himself? A woman in his life, finally?* "Which friend has news?"

"Remember Ahmed Mohammed? He's been with the Hempstead Institute since he left here. His group just got FDA approval for an antibiotic they developed." Akira's voice rose with excitement. "This is a true breakthrough drug, effective against most resistant organisms in postop patients. Once it's manufactured, it'll be a godsend for patients with rare hospital-acquired infections, such as methicillin resistant staphylococcus aureus."

"That's fantastic! Wow! So happy for Ahmed. What's the next step?"

"Well, hard to believe, but there are problems getting someone to produce it. It's cheap to make, that's not the issue. The problem is that it's only given intravenously, and it isn't for everyday infections like tonsillitis or ear infections. So, it's not a moneymaker for drug companies.

Mohammed's not sure who'll take it up. But I think he recently got a lead."

"Surely somebody will make it," Tom said, his naivete and idealism both on display. "Such a meaningful contribution to science. Ahmed must be so proud."

"I'm sure he is, but you know how humble he is. He'd never let on that he's proud. He says it's all 'Allah's will,' attributes all his success to God."

"What's the drug's name?"

"Right now, they call it by its experimental name: X2470. I don't know a generic name," Akira said. "Tom, I'm sorry, but I'm late for another meeting, bane of my existence. Let's get together, soon. Email me when you have time, and I'll get back to you. Good talking to you."

"After your meeting, can you email me Ahmed's contact information? I need to reconnect with him."

***

Tom remembered Ahmed Mohammed fondly. When they first met, Tom had just returned from the Middle East War, where Muslims were enemy combatants. Initially, he had to admit, he had an implicit bias against this Muslim pharmacologist. But once he knew him better, prejudice dissolved, and he was grateful Ahmed was on the Zylinski team. It was Ahmed who first suggested someone was probably tampering with the PTSD drug in the study. His suspicion led to solving who was doing it and why. Tom called and left a message on Ahmed's service.

***

"You have a bunch of messages," Dolores said, hurrying into his office. "Want them now?"

"Yeah, good a time as any."

He handed some calls off to a volunteer. However, one call was particularly interesting. A medical student at Brown University had stumbled onto his website and was excited with the mission of PharmaTruth and wanted to get involved. Tom punched in the number.

"Hi, this is Max."

"Uh, hello." Tom was surprised by the quick answer. "This is Tom Barrett from PharmaTruth, returning your call."

"Jesus, the head guy!" Max exclaimed. "Didn't expect this. This is so cool, talking to you."

He must think I'm a lot older than I am. Tom was amused he was being idolized by a millennial. He liked him instantly, not because of that flattering comment, but because he was so guileless and open. Tom identified with him, recalling his own medical student days when life was newer and simpler. "So, what can I do for you?"

"Well, I'm not really sure, ya know? I'm totally against pharmaceutical behemoths. I'd like to know how I can get involved with your – what should I call it – agency?"

"Not really an agency; that sounds governmental. We're a private non-profit corporation. Have a particular way you'd like to help?" Tom said, not knowing what to say to this kid with no concrete goal, only animus for drug companies.

"So, we have this public health course, ya know, and our instructor told us to figure out a project, anything, to advance consumers' stakes in health care. We have all year to do this while we go to classes like biochemistry and physiology," Max said.

"You're in second year, right?"

"Yeah. Actually, this public health course is the one I'm most interested in. Biochemistry I had in college and physiology too. And, uh, there's another guy who might partner with me. Name's Casey Andrews."

Tom was getting good vibes from Max.

"Why don't you come talk with me. Bring your friend. Maybe we can work something out."

"Awesome! I'll talk to him and call you back. Thanks!"

How can I make these two young idealists useful to PharmaTruth while they learn something valuable? All I remember when I was a medical student listening to boring public health lectures, was Professor Werner, his thick Viennese accent extolling the virtues of sewers. Dull public health courses, dealing with abstractions had no cache for students.

Surgery was sexier, and internal medicine was what the smart ones chose. Movies and television depict overworked residents (usually hunks needing haircuts and shaves), and doctors dramatically saving individual lives every day. Most medical students scoffed at non-remunerative public health careers that merely ensure healthy water and provide immunizations to large populations. But that was before Legionnaire's disease, lead poisoning, HIV, Ebola, influenza, opioid addiction and COVID-19 epidemics all captured world-wide attention. Maybe things are different now. Young, enthusiastic, and cause-oriented students have often been a stimulus for great ideas.

Tom smiled as he contemplated having contact once more with students in medical training, always a source of energy. But questions remained: how could he involve them for *their* benefit while helping PharmaTruth?

Dolores interrupted his reverie, handing Tom a slip of paper.

"Here's a message from a Colonel Higgins. Didn't know who he was but he sounded like he knew you," she said.

Tom sat up quickly and reached for the message.

"Yes, I know him. He was my CO in Iraq. I was expecting his call."

Chapter 10

"That's so great Colonel," Tom said, once he was connected. "When do you have time to meet with Katharine and me?"

"Drop the Colonel, Tom. We've been through too much together to be formal. My time is real free. It depends on the two of you. I think mostly you since you're on the other side of the country."

"I'll call Katharine. As I look at my calendar, I can come this week. After that it gets more crowded. Could we meet in the evening at the Sheraton opposite the airport?"

***

The flight to San Diego took off at dawn, but it was the only non-stop Tom could get. He'd arranged to meet Katharine at the Sheraton around five. Ben Higgins would arrive for dinner at six. He used the day to go to Balboa Park and wander through the museums and the conservatory before going to the hotel for dinner.

Katharine was an enchanting sight striding toward him with her engaging smile and her outstretched arms. A warm flush spread over his face and his heart rate quickened. He was again surprised at how she affected him, but then, why not? She was a lovely woman.

"So glad to see you," she said as they hugged. Her familiar scent flooded Tom's senses, and her warm body had its effect as they embraced. "Thank you for coming," she said. "And for getting Colonel Higgins to meet with me. I can't thank you enough."

"It's a good excuse to see you again," Tom said, immediately embarrassed by the truth of what he'd just said. "I'm happy that Colonel Higgins lives nearby and can join us. Want to grab a drink?"

They found a table near the large window looking out over the bay and ordered drinks.

"Are you staying here tonight?" Katharine asked.

"Yes, got an early flight back in the morning. A lot going on back at PharmaTruth."

"Wanna tell me about it?"

"No, I'd rather talk about you. What's going on in your life?"

"Not much new. I feel a lot better after our talk. I know talking to Colonel Higgins will help too. Thank you so much for arranging this. Danny was right about you."

Tom had his usual problem accepting compliments, so he let this comment pass without response.

"How are the boys?" Tom knew this question was perfunctory and her answer would be also.

"They're doing okay, thanks."

So much emotional uncertainty hung in the air over their heads; feelings of loss about Danny and the palpable but unspoken sexual tension between them. The conversation stagnated until Tom felt compelled to speak honestly.

"Katharine, I'm going to be frank with you. I find you very attractive. That makes me feel guilty because our connection to each other is Danny. Can we talk about this?"

Katharine scooted her chair closer to the table, clasped her hands together around the stem of her glass.

"Yes, I'd like to sweep away this barrier. I loved Danny as much as anyone can love another person. I miss him every day. I will never forget him. He's the father of my children and I see him in each of them in different ways." She looked intently at Tom. "I find you attractive too. You're very much like Danny, maybe that's why you two got so close so fast, and I have to admit that I sometimes fantasize about you. I feel guilty about that too, but that makes me angry. I've lost the love of my life and my best friend. But I'm still young. Do I have to feel lonely the rest of my life?"

"Maybe my telling you I witnessed Danny's death and Colonel Higgins showing you precisely where he died will allow you to move away from that terrible event." He reached across the table and took her hand in his. "No, you shouldn't feel lonely for years into the future. You should have the chance for happiness. This doesn't mean forgetting Danny. You'll never do that.

"But I have to say something else. It would be easy for me to invite you to spend the night with me. If you accepted, it would transform a friendship into a love affair that would always carry the phantom of Danny with it. I worry that wouldn't allow it to flourish."

"I've thought about that." She looked down at the table. "You're right, unfortunately. If we'd met under different circumstances, I think it would have been easy for us to fall for one another."

They fell silent, both absorbed in variations of what might have been.

Tom rose, came around the table, pulled her up from her chair and they stood in each other's arms.

Before long, they were greeted by the booming voice of Ben Higgins.

"Damn good thing I got here!" he joked. They both turned, grinned like school kids, and Tom introduced Colonel Higgins to Katharine.

Higgins set a brief case on the floor next to the table. A waiter appeared and asked if they wanted to eat at this table.

"No reason to move," Tom said.

"So good to meet you, Katharine. I'm sorry it's like this but I'm hoping I can be of some consolation to you," Higgins said in a reassuring voice.

"Thanks for taking the trouble to help with this. It may be silly, but it seems important." she said.

"Not silly at all. I've had this same request from several people," Higgins said.

After dinner, Higgins dug into his briefcase and produced a map and a sheaf of papers.

"I've gone through these papers that give the geographical coordinates of our field hospital. I've used these coordinates to tell you with considerable accuracy that the spot marked in red on this map is precisely where our hospital operating room was when the blast occurred. It follows that this is the site of Danny's death.

"Tom mentioned you asked about going there. I would strongly advise you not to try. It's dangerous even getting to Iraq. To get to this godforsaken place would require getting a military truck, and I know the military would not provide that for your purpose. The chances of getting there safely are slim to none."

Katharine looked at the map carefully and held the pages Higgins gave her with shaking hands and reverence.

"Colonel Higgins, I'm so thankful for your doing this for me. I think just having this information, and especially the map, may be enough. I agree a trip there is a fool's errand. I'd already decided I wouldn't try to do it."

The waiter came with the bill for the meal, signaling the end of their meeting. Tom accepted the check after protestations from both. Exchanging glances Tom and Higgins pushed back their chairs and stood up, looking at Katharine. She rose with tears in her eyes, hugged both men, thanking them for their support, then turned to leave. Tom didn't want Ben Higgins to notice the tears in his eyes. He stepped back and watched her shapely body, her long brown shining hair and long legs move away from them, her fragrance trailing behind her, probably out of his life. *Was I wrong to stop anything from even starting? Will I ever see her again?*

Chapter 11

Back in Boston a couple of days later, Tom's phone rang. "Dr. Barrett? This is Ahmed Mohammed returning your call. So good to hear your voice again! I hope you're well."

"It's Tom, for heaven's sake! I'm well, thanks. Say, I heard from Akira that you've had great success! Tell me about it."

"Very exciting." After telling him the whole story, Ahmed said, "We couldn't find any one to produce it until yesterday. A drug company called 'Pylea,' right here in Cambridge, is interested."

"You hold a patent on it?"

"Yes...well, Hempstead, where I work, does."

"Know anything about Pylea?"

"Nothing. Their website is 'under construction,' but it was recently bought by a Mr. Reginald Warner, who's both the owner and CEO. I'll find out more when I meet with him next week."

"You have a lawyer?" Tom asked, red flags going up.

"Um, no, not personally, but Hempstead, my employer, is sending their property rights specialist with me. Don't worry, no one is going to pull the wool over our eyes. Remember, I was the most suspicious about our adventure with nepenthe at Zylinski."

"You were, at that. Can you send me your publication on the new drug? I'd like to know the science behind it."

"It's in an email as we speak. I'd love your feedback. I have to go. I'll let you know how my meeting goes with Mr. Warner."

***

Tuesday came and shortly before two, all the interested parties gathered at Pylea Pharmaceutical Company's office in Cambridge. Ahmed Mohammed and his associate, Jordan Gundersen, were ushered into a conference room overlooking the Charles River. Warner, Shelby, and Bernie Steinmetz were on one side of the table and Ahmed and Gundersen on the other. Coffee was offered with no takers.

"Welcome, Dr. Mohammed and Mr. Gundersen. We're so pleased ya'll could come to discuss your new drug," Warner said, exuding charm and good will in a heavy west Texas drawl.

"Thank you for having us," Ahmed said in his low quiet voice.

"We're very interested in your drug, Doctor. This could be a lifesaver for so many people. I understand it's not that difficult to fabricate."

"That's right, sir. It's a simple compound. I'm surprised it hadn't been discovered before," Ahmed said.

"Once we've taken care of all the usual paperwork – Bernie can work with you, Mr. Gundersen – are you a lawyer?"

"I'm a lawyer, yes, but my job description is property rights manager," Gundersen said. "Our legal department will get involved as we move forward."

"Who has the patent? You?" Warner nodded to Ahmed. "Or Hempstead?"

"Hempstead."

"Well, Bernie, talk with Gundersen, get this deal done. I think we can get the medication under production quickly," Warner said. "I bought this here company a few weeks ago and this drug will let us hit the ground running. We're so excited to help patients, you know, that's our number one goal here. With more resistant organisms popping up every day, especially after operations, this drug will fill a gaping hole in our treatment stable. Maybe it will even convince me to go ahead with a hip replacement," he said with a smile.

"What does Pylea have in mind for pricing?" Ahmed asked in a near whisper.

"We're working on that," Warner replied. "Still in the works. I'll let you know when we're further along."

"Perhaps our next step would be for me to meet with your lawyer to work out the business arrangements," Gundersen suggested. "I think we're eager to get this on the market, as you apparently are. It looks like we're all on the same page. Devil's always in the details."

"Okay, we'll set up times to go over those 'devils' and come up, quickly I hope, with a contract acceptable to both sides," Steinmetz said.

"I've always believed short meetings are best," Warner said. "If there's nothing else to discuss, let's let these smart contract guys get their heads together and get this show on the road."

With that, Warner stood up and headed to the door, waving graciously to Ahmed as he left. He pulled a cigarette from his pocket, and had it lit before he disappeared into his office. Within minutes, Shelby was with him.

"That Mohammed boy's naïve, ya think?" Warner said to Shelby. "I think we can do whatever we want with him. Is he Muslim? He sure is dark lookin."

"I think with the name Mohammed, he's Muslim," Shelby said without betraying a trace of incredulity that Warner had asked such a question. He'd learned the hard way not to respond when his boss uttered bigoted perspectives or asked dimwitted questions. Once, Warner had pushed him hard against a wall when he challenged him. Since that day, he handled his volatile and impetuous employer with the kind of patience usually reserved for oppositional four-year-old children.

"Well, once we get the contract, we'll market it like hell. And we're gonna price it real high because it'll be in huge demand at every hospital," Warner said. "We'll say the high price is because of how much research and development was necessary; what we always say. The hospitals will have to stock it, and our job'll be to make damn sure the great unwashed out there – otherwise known as patients – believe they can't trust any hospital that doesn't have it.

"We're gonna get insurance companies on board, too. Concentrate on big ones, I know a lot of them, and I can lean on them to pay. They know I know their dirty little secrets. Small insurance companies won't be able to pay what we're gonna charge, but fuck 'em and their stupid subscribers who don't know enough to shop around."

Warner lit another cigarette, went to his liquor cabinet and pulled out his favorite bourbon. He poured a generous glass for himself, not offering any to Shelby, and propped his feet on his desk. "I'll be rich! I'll sell this company for big bucks and spend my life with some bimbo on a beach in the Caribbean."

"What if insurance companies balk at paying?" Shelby asked with temerity.

"They won't dare!" Warner roared, his face flushing, jerking his feet off his desk and facing Shelby. "No chance!"

Shelby backed off, changed the subject.

"You're gonna need someone with professional credentials to organize our promotional campaign. We'll also need an army of detail people to make the rounds of big hospitals," Shelby said. "I'll get cracking on advertising for a doctor or nurse who can help us with that first part. How shall we recruit a sales force?"

"I'll call salespeople who used to work for me. They'll have ideas about recruiting more," Warner said. "Salespeople are easy to find. They move from one company to another, whoever's offering higher commissions. With this drug's high price, the commission's gonna be huge. You can always buy salesmen. And get some girl sales reps. They're appealing to hospitals who think that a company that hires girls is progressive. Besides, I like having good lookin' girls around."

***

Ahmed and Jordan walked back to their office, a few blocks away.

"What'd you think?" Gundersen asked.

"Warner seemed in a hurry. A crude man. On the other hand, no one else has evinced any interest," Ahmed said. "Let's work out the legal details carefully and proceed. We need to watch Mr. Reginald Warner closely. There's something about him that my ethics radar picked up on. He dodged the question about cost. That worries me a little. But if we proceed cautiously, I think we'll be okay. What did you think?"

"Pretty much the same. I agree we need to watch our step. We hold Cidal's patent, and as long as we get a fair percentage of the profit, I think we'll be okay."

"I'm going to talk with Tom Barrett about this. He's running a non-profit that scrutinizes questionable business practices of pharma companies. Pylea could be his private little petri dish to watch one company's behavior."

Chapter 12

"Pylea Pharmaceuticals. Karen speaking. May I help you?"

"I'm calling about the pharmacologist job you advertised," Dina said. "Is it still available?"

"Yes, it's still open. I'm Karen, Head of Human Resources. Why don't you come in, and we can tell you all about it?"

"When do you have time available?"

"How would next Tuesday, around 9, be for you?"

"Yes, that works. Should I send you my resume and references?"

"Yes, please email them. We won't contact your references until after our personal interview. See you on Tuesday."

Walking into Pylea Pharmaceuticals, Dina had a sudden rush of doubt. *What am I doing here?* Her eyes darted around, taking in the cold steel and glass building. An army of strangers poured into her consciousness. Her stomach churned as she poked the elevator button, stepped in, and went to the eighth floor.

"Your curriculum vitae is very impressive: BS in nursing, PhD in pharmacology, lecturer at the nursing school," Karen said. "Why would you want to give all that up?"

The right question. Why would I? Dina considered her answer before responding.

"Well, I've read about your new antibiotic, and the pharmacologist in me is intrigued and fascinated by its potential. This is truly an exciting breakthrough drug. At a personal level, my mother died recently, triggered by a methicillin resistant infection. I have both a professional and personal interest in seeing this drug succeed."

"Oh, I am sorry," Karen said. "My heart goes out to you." She paused for a moment. "I showed your CV to Mr. Warner, our CEO. He was struck by your background and wants to talk to you. He's committed to getting this drug on the market quickly and needs the kind of expertise you have to help introduce it. Let me see if he's available."

Dina was shown into Reginald Warner's office. After getting over her surprise at getting a face-to-face interview with the head man, she surveyed the office. Her eyes moved over his massive oak desk with a high-back leather chair and a floor-to-ceiling window overlooking the Charles River. His receptionist motioned to one of two smaller leather-bound chairs in front of his desk. The pungent odor of cigarette smoke hung in the air. At the nursing school there was a "Strictly No Smoking" rule on the whole campus. It seemed incongruent that a company in the business of restoring people to good health would allow smoking. And this was the CEO's office.

Moments later, Warner came in from a side door and strode toward Dina. She stood up, and he welcomed her with a broad smile.

At five-feet-nine, she was slightly taller than Warner. Her black hair reached below her shoulders. Full cheeks set below dark eyes framed a petite nose. Her generous lips drew attention away from a thyroid surgery scar on her long neck.

"So glad to meet you, Doctor. Karen showed me your great credentials," he said. As he shook her hand, Dina noticed his eyes scanning her from head to toe, his eyes stopping momentarily on her breasts.

"Have a seat," Warner said.

He watched her closely as she sat and crossed her legs. Dina was mildly uncomfortable but dismissed his scrutiny as the typical thing that men do.

"So, what do you know about our new drug?" Warner began.

"I've read the original paper by Dr. Mohammed and what's on your website. It sounds like an important agent."

"Oh, yeah, it's important. Hugely important. It'll revolutionize the treatment of post-op infections from bad bugs."

Dina involuntarily swept her hair back from her eyes, an old nervous habit, as she took in his declarative manner of speaking.

"Can you give me an idea what this job would entail?" Dina said, filling an awkward pause as he continued to look at her.

"Sorta up to y'all. I need someone who knows about drugs to keep us from claiming things we shouldn't and to tell us the best way to say the things we should."

"I'd need time to study the drug and its development to do that, but it's something I'm interested in," Dina said. She still felt confused about what this man was looking for. He seemed glib and superficial in describing what qualifications he wanted in someone who'd be assessing the merits of this "hugely important" drug.

"When could you start?" Warner asked abruptly.

Astounded by this precipitous offering of an important job, she stammered, "We – we, well, we haven't even talked about salary or benefits. Can you tell me about that?"

"Minor details," he laughed. He floated a proposal, and she was stunned.

"That's very generous," she said. "I'm surprised by an offer like that. You don't know much about me."

"I've been at this business a long time. I know quality when I see it. It's where I trust my gut. When you work here, one thing you'll learn about me is that I make decisions quick, and I'm almost always right. I'm offering this job to you and hope you can make a quick decision too."

"How quickly?"

"I like how you think! Direct and to the point. How 'bout in the next 24 hours?"

"Um…I need to consider this," Dina managed to say, not knowing how else to respond to this impetuous man. "I'll call tomorrow, okay?"

"Great! I know you won't regret working for me. I'll see to it that you enjoy your work." He winked. With that, he stood up, offered his hand to her and left the room, reaching into his pocket for a cigarette.

Flustered by the speed of the interview, the offer of a new job, and a major increase in salary, she dropped her purse on the floor. As she was picking it up, Karen came in carrying a folder.

"These are the forms you need to fill out when you decide to take the job. Mr. Warner said you'd call tomorrow. You can call me, and we'll take it from there."

"Thanks, Karen. Talk to you tomorrow." Dina noted her use of 'when' not 'if.'

"Sure hope you join us!" Karen said in her perky voice.

After a sleepless night, Dina decided. The mission seemed right, and the pay was fantastic. *What's not to like? Well, Warner was a little weird, but he probably won't be around much once I'm working. Wish I knew more about other people working there – what their backgrounds are, what they're like as people, what made them join the company, but that's probably going to have to come later.*

***

"Wonderful!" said Karen, when Dina called and accepted the offer. "When can you begin workin'?"

"I need to give notice to the nursing school. How about two weeks from Monday?"

"This is great news. Can't wait for you to begin. I'll get an office set up for you."

Saying goodbye to her friends at the nursing school was poignant. She'd been there several years and hadn't had more than a few bad days. Her boss had been tough but fair and her coworkers a pleasure to be around. She'd had carte blanche on her projects, but she'd never had a burning sense of mission. She hoped her new job would stoke that passion.

On her first day at Pylea, Karen led her to an office right next to Warner's, a little surprising. She'd had uncomfortable vibes about him since her interview and wished she were further away. But she put aside these misgivings, dug right in and spent her time learning everything about Cidal from its inception through its clinical trials, primarily from Dr. Mohammed's publications. In those rare moments when she wasn't studying Cidal, she huddled with other department heads, all members of the so-called "Executive Council." They met every Monday morning, and in these meetings, Dina became comfortable that Pylea had capable staff and was well organized. Warner ran these meetings briskly and professionally, a different picture of him than when she first met him. Maybe her apprehensions were groundless. He clearly knew how to lead, and he'd assembled a skilled management team.

One morning as the council meeting was ending, Warner asked her to come to his office. Dina didn't think she'd done or said anything that would lead to his disapproval but being asked to his office made her nervous.

"Come in, Dina," he said warmly. "Part of my management technique is to have private meetings with council members from time to time. I waited to meet with you until you'd had a chance to get used to this place.

"How's it going? You settling in okay? Anything you need?"

Dina relaxed. *Just a routine meeting with the boss who's checking a new employee's adjustment to a new job, right?*

"Doing well. In fact, very well. The more I learn about Cidal, the more impressed I am. And Dr. Mohammed's work is a real breakthrough. Someday I'd like to meet him."

"That can be arranged. He doesn't come here often but next time he does, I'll see that you meet him.

"Come over to the window. I want to point out one of the pleasures of being on the Charles River."

Dina walked over beside Warner as he pointed to a crew in a scull, practicing for running in the October Head of the Charles Regatta.

"Now, where I grew up, that kind of sport was considered sissified. We played a lot of football, not that touch football stuff the Kennedys used to play down on the Cape, but real tackle football.

"Where did you grow up?" Dina asked, trying to enter into a friendly conversation.

"West Texas, small town you never heard of. But here I am, owner of a big pharmaceutical company about to introduce the most important drug to come along in years. And our office is located smack-dab in the People's Republic of Cambridge, seat of left-wing liberality in the U.S. of A."

As he said this, he slid his hand across Dina's back, ostensibly to improve her view of the boat. She wasn't sure what she should do, but she didn't want to over-react. An unwarranted and uninvited touch by a man she hardly knew and who exercised quite a lot of power over her was an invasion of her private space, exactly the thing the MeToo movement had been organized to oppose.

"Look at that!" she said excitedly, pointing to a speedboat going too fast and too close to the scull, taking this opportunity to move away from Warner's hand. "That maniac could capsize the scull!"

Warner laughed.

Did he know it was an excuse to pull away from his advance? Dina took a slow breath to calm herself.

"I'm glad you're liking your new job," Warner said. "I hope we can get to know each other better over time. See you tomorrow."

Dina went back to her office. Her hands shook as she picked up papers on her desk. *Is this the opening gambit of a pattern? Have I made an enormous mistake?* She sighed and sat staring at her computer, trying to focus on work and rid herself of apprehension. *Who can I talk to about it? Karen, in*

Human Resources? No, hardly know her, and she wouldn't want to hear anything about the boss, she's obviously a company woman. It had been several years since Dina had worked in a male-dominated workplace. The nursing school, with few exceptions, was female; this kind of encounter didn't happen there. Her skills at countering unwanted advances had rusted away. She just hoped this behavior didn't progress.

***

In Monday morning's meeting with the Executive Council, Warner passed out a short simple agenda: pricing Cidal.

"As you see from the agenda our meeting today will be brief. This item is of utmost importance and appropriate pricing of Cidal will ensure our success. I've determined that we'll bundle the cost of the drug and its delivery system into a $500,000 complete, start-to-finish treatment package. I've already made this decision, so this is an information session, not a discussion."

Stunned silence followed Warner's pronouncement. The council members stared at the table, averting their gazes from Warner and from each other. No one knew what to say. No one moved.

Dina was similarly shocked. *This is extraordinary, his simply dictating pricing of Cidal. What's the point of having this council, if major decisions like this are top down, with no input, even from the financial people? My opinion about pricing is irrelevant; I'm a scientist, not a bean counter, but not to ask his associates is outrageous. Who is this guy? What are his goals?*

"I take it from the lack of comments that you all agree, so the meeting is adjourned. Have a good day!" Warner said. He left the room, reaching predictively for a cigarette.

"$500,000 per treatment? Unbelievable!" said Curt Neuffer, the Chief Financial Officer.

"That's gonna be a hard sell to hospitals and insurance companies. I hope he knows what he's doing. I wonder how he came up with that figure."

"He pulled it out of the ether," said Paul Burrer, Director of Marketing. "A hard sell is an understatement. Unless he has a sweetheart deal with major insurance companies, that figure won't fly. Adverse publicity alone will make our job impossible."

"Other companies are doing the same thing, for chrissake," Peter Snavely said. "When I was with Reggie at Drum Pharmaceuticals in Texas, we were astounded when the whole EpiPen pricing brouhaha came up. But you know what happened -- that completely blew over. The public's interest in this stuff flags over time. Other drug houses are raising prices all over the country. So why shouldn't we cash in on this bonanza? There's big money to be made so we should hop on this gravytrain."

Dina kept her mouth shut even as she was appalled at Snavely's callousness. Warner and Snavely were clearly of the same mind. Who else from the Executive Council was with them? Time to be circumspect. So depressing and worrisome that this company she'd just joined with such high hopes was heading in a direction she considered unethical, maybe even immoral.

When she got home, she wanted distraction. Her work world was in upheaval, and she needed an escape. She turned on the television, which depressed her even more:

inane commercials, national and international leaders lying about their policies and intents, and incessant football games interrupted only by truck and beer commercials.

Maybe if she did research on drug delivery systems, she could calm down and gain perspective. Typing "pharmaceuticals" on the search bar, she clicked on her browser. Scrolling through the topic list, she stumbled onto a website called "PharmaTruth." *Now there's an oxymoron, if ever I've seen one.* She opened the website and her interest perked up.

PharmaTruth
Our Mission: Shine a Light on Questionable
Practices of Pharmaceutical Companies.

**This free website is here as an information
exchange between our staff and real people who
have had difficulty obtaining drugs because:**
Drugs are priced out of your reach.
Your insurance is insufficient for payment.

"Drugs priced out your reach." That's exactly what Cidal would be, if it went on the market for what Warner was proposing.

"Your insurance is insufficient for payment." Surely that would be true, unless Warner has a Merlin-like influence over insurance companies. Is that likely? He's far up the ladder in the industry. He obviously has influence, but with insurers?

Dare I contact this website? What if Warner found out? But how would he know? Would contacting them be confidential? It would be on my personal computer, but that could be hacked if anyone wanted to find out what I'm doing. Maybe I should do it on the library computer. I can't believe such an organization exists. Are they *to be trusted? What if someone finds out I've gone to their website? Would I lose my job? Whistleblowers become pariahs in whatever business they've been in. Some are threatened, harassed. Could I get hurt? Debbie? This is taking a big chance.*

Chapter 13

"Nelsons has such a profound grasp of Shostakovich," Cynthia said as they left Tanglewood. "And I love how his body dances with the music." She was in high spirits as they rushed into the Richmond Inn, tore their clothes off and had glorious sex in the four-poster bed. "I love you so much; I hope this lasts forever."

Tom woke from this provocative and arousing dream about times gone by. He turned over and tried to go back to sleep to dial into it again. He wished Cynthia were there to be touched and held. But then he looked and saw it was seven AM. He was due in for a board meeting at eight. Hustling out of bed, he jumped into the shower.

While jogging to his office, his mind flew back to Cynthia.

I should call her. That was the deal we agreed to, that we'd get together occasionally to see what happens. Do I want anything to"happen?" If dreams uncover our unconscious desires, then maybe I do. Fond memories are there, sure, but what followed put a toxic stain on the relationship. Is there anything that can dissolve that stain? I just don't know. But I should call her. I promised.

He arrived at PharmaTruth in time for his meeting. Flipping through a pile of messages, he noticed one from Max Schorr. He'd call him after the meeting.

"We've gotten a pile of responses to our website," Dolores said. "Pretty amazing that so many folks have stories to tell about problems with drug companies. Makes this place an important agency for change."

"Only if we go about it correctly," said David Longstreet. "As a lawyer, I want to build a strong case, get prominent Congress people interested in holding hearings and passing new legislation. Only that will begin to correct these practices. Drug companies won't change because of their great moral compasses."

"I agree with that, even though I've represented drug houses," said Francis Boyle. "You gotta remember these cats get paid for making sure their companies make substantial profits. Stocks only go up if their profits go up. It's capitalism, after all. Never mind that people's lives are involved. They argue that they're offering a product just like hospitals, food companies, car companies, etcetera. They don't see themselves as social service agencies, that's for sure."

Tom felt satisfied that he'd seen an emerging consensus among the board members. He was encouraged that team consolidation was taking place. His mind returned to Cynthia, and he followed through with his earlier intention.

"Cyn, this is Tom. I want to set a time for our next – what should I call it? – date. I thought maybe we could go to the symphony or a Celtics game. Gimme a call."

His next call was to Max.

"Hi Max, Tom Barrett here. When can we meet?"

"You call it," Max said in his breezy manner. "Our public health course is open-ended. We have lots of research time to spend in the library."

"When can your friend Casey come? Same as you?"

"Oh, yeah. Tell me when you want us, we'll be there."

"How about this afternoon? Around two?"

"Done. See you then. Any special instructions about getting past security in your building?"

"I'll leave word at the security desk. Just identify yourselves and they'll tell you how to find our office."

Max looked pretty much as Tom had imagined: medium height; ample black curly hair; a scruffy, short black beard; and a wiry frame. In college, a soccer ball had bashed in his nose, and it was angled slightly toward his left ear. It only enhanced rugged good looks. His friend, Casey Andrews, was taller, with a fair complexion and smooth face. In fact, it didn't look like he *could* grow a beard. His strawberry blond hair and blue eyes were a contrast to Max's coloration. His broad smile made him look like a Kennedy brother.

"Welcome to PharmaTruth. We need to figure out what you guys can do for us and what we can do for you. Does your public health course have any parameters for your project?"

"You know of any guidelines?" Max said, leaning towards Casey.

"We have to adhere to a protocol for writing it up, but it's pretty much a blank slate as far as designing the project."

"Let's start by having you field website hits and see where that leads. I have in mind the possibility of your doing interviews of leads that come in. It'll be important figuring out who's legit or not, and then documenting what may become the catalyst for an investigation or exposé. How's that sound?"

"Good, worthwhile," Max said.

"Casey?"

"Okay by me. When do we start?"

Tom walked them down the hall and introduced them to Leila, the volunteer coordinator. Her eyes lit up when she saw the two young studs. A spirited conversation filled the volunteer room as she led them to places on the website control desk.

Tom felt satisfied that action was beginning. *I think this is gonna be great.*

***

"Let me tell you what I've been doing and get your advice," Tom said as he and Cynthia found seats at the Garden for the Celts game. "I took on a couple of med students to interview responders to our website. I'm trying to decide how they should conduct these interviews. Think they should do it by phone?"

"Huh? You expect me to answer that? I don't have a clue!"

"Yeah, dumb question. I'm really asking myself. But you were always a good brain-storming partner. I'm trying to figure how to use these guys. Maybe, you know, if they could screen the calls and then what?"

"Why not use a medical model? Remember that? Med students are assigned to take histories and do exams on patients and present their findings to a preceptor. After a preceptor checks on the patient, student and preceptor discuss it. So, using this model, you'd create a template for the type of information you're fairly sure will pan out. Like identifying symptoms of disease, you'd be collecting website messages and deciding together which people the students should talk to. After they interview them, meet again and discuss what they learned."

"See why I asked you? Cyn, you're brilliant. I remember now why I admired you so much in our emergency department back then."

"It seems like a different epoch, doesn't it? So much has gone down since then. Oh, look, here comes the team. Who are we playing tonight?"

After the game they went to Remy's bar for a snack and a beer. Tom laughed more than he had in months. He put aside his serious role of leading a non-profit to dig into dark corners of corporate life in America. Cynthia was also in a felicitous and playful mood, happy to forget she was dean of a nursing school. They bantered about each other's faults and at times stopped to look at one another in a familiar way.

"It's eleven-thirty. I'd better head home," Cynthia said. "Look outside, it's snowing! That wasn't in the forecast."

"You still believe those weather people? I look outside, put my finger in the air, and usually know what's gonna happen." Tom stared into his beer, his mood changing from light-hearted to serious. "I...I" he stammered. "I think you should stay at my place tonight. You shouldn't drive back in this snowstorm. I have a spare room." Looking up, he saw the confused look on Cyn's face. "It's not like we haven't slept under the same roof before," he said, trying to read her reaction. Her elbows were on the bar, chin resting on her upturned palms, eyes fixed on the bottles against the wall.

"You know, I can drive back to Worcester, no problem. I've done it many times. This little bit of snow doesn't bother me. I have 4-wheel drive. It's not that late, no big deal," she yammered on, all the time keeping her gaze on the stacked bottles.

"Methinks the lady doth protest too much," Tom said after a few moments' pause. Both were perplexed at this critical fork in the road and neither knew which branch to take. If she didn't accept his invitation, it could be the end of their newfound friendship, or whatever this dance of theirs was called. If she accepted, would it lead to their falling into bed, allowing the passion of sex to determine their future?

"No big deal is right," Tom said. "We're sitting here, scared shitless about the significance of everything we say and do. We both need to chill out, relax, and stop worrying like a couple of teenagers about what it will mean if we spend a night in the same apartment. Come with me, let's take our chances. We've both faced much bigger challenges than this, so why are we being such wimps?"

"I don't want to hear how I finagled you into this," Cynthia said with a smile. "In olden days, social mores demanded that damsels were never to be forward or seductive. Lonely heroines spent their lives regretting a man who got away because they were afraid to offer themselves. Times have changed, but now we go to shrinks when we woo a man only to lose him later."

"You're reading the wrong books," Tom laughed. "While those uptight damsels in Austen novels were losing their men, the peasants were out in the fields fucking their brains out. Let's go to my apartment and stop agonizing."

By midnight they were safely ensconced in Tom's condo. Cynthia looked around, her eyes landing on a couple of unframed paintings leaning against the living room wall.

"Nice paintings. Look original. When did you start collecting art?"

Tom flushed, scratched his head, and said, "I painted those myself."

"Really? When did you start that hobby?"

"I wanted to sculpt but it's hard with only one flipper. The art teacher suggested I try painting. Turns out, I'm not too bad. She started me off with still life and now, as you can see, I'm doing some abstract stuff. It puts my mind in a different place. Really enjoying it."

"Well. A surgeon with a right brain that works. What do you know? These are quite good.

"Got an extra toothbrush? How 'bout a change of clothes?" she chuckled, turning back to Tom and slipping off her coat. "This proves I didn't have an ulterior motive tonight."

"Will you stop? You must have a guilty conscience, or you wouldn't keep bringing this up." Tom smiled as he spoke. "You can sleep in one of my shirts, or naked, your choice. I'd rather sleep with you naked."

With that invitation, a decision was reached, and they did what both were aching to do.

***

In the morning, Tom rose before Cynthia and cooked fried eggs, made toast. He brought the tray up to Cynthia in bed, also loaded with orange juice, raspberries, blueberries, and steaming black, dark-roast coffee.

"You are something," Cynthia said, happily surprised. "Don't remember this kind of service before. Do you usually keep fresh fruit or were you always planning on having your way with me last night?"

"Of course, you know what a horny guy I am," Tom said, grinning as he sat down on the bed beside her. "Actually, I've become a pretty good grocery shopper and cook. I know how to live well by myself, but I'd rather have someone else to share my life with."

He looked away, embarrassed that these words escaped. But he continued with this thread.

"Let's just say I'm reasonably happy with my life. PharmaTruth has given me purpose and keeps me furiously busy. In moments of reflection, though, I wonder what it'd be like living the life I thought I'd have. You know, wife, kids, dogs, soccer games, suburbia, vacations."

"I fantasize about that rosy scenario, too," Cynthia said. "But when I see several friends who've tried it, they don't seem blissfully happy, some had ugly divorces and post-divorce poverty. That's removed the scales from my eyes. My divorce from Dirk was so amicable -- luckily no kids -- I consider myself the exception."

"So, what is the answer to the age-old philosophical question of the meaning of life?" Tom asked. "I read a funny book by Dan Klein. You know, that Harvard philosopher slash comedian who says that every time he finds the meaning of life, they change it."

"The hedonists might have had it right -- do what feels good, often as possible."

"Yeah, we're such good examples of that," Tom said sardonically. "But we should allow ourselves a little hedonism. Like last night.

"Hey," he continued. "Let's plan a weekend trip someplace. Winter's almost here. I can't ski, and I think a weekend in the Caribbean sounds better anyway. What do you think?"

"Lying on a beach in the Bahamas sounds lovely. Shall I book it?"

"Does the weekend after next work for you?"

"Think so. I'll let you know," Cynthia said. She smiled warmly at him.

"What're you doing the rest of today? It's Saturday. We could go to a museum or something," Tom said. "See some real art."

"I need to get some fresh clothes at home. Ever been to the Worcester Art Museum? We could do that, spend the day in Worcester. I know of a great Thai restaurant there. And if you feel inclined, you could see what I've done with my pad in Worcester, even stay the night."

"I like it. Let's get going," Tom said. *Okay, taking the plunge. Hopefully it was a swim and not sink situation.*

Chapter 14

Max and Casey stared at their laptops, scrolling through hits on the PharmaTruth website.

"Case, look at this one," Max called out.

'I'd like more information on PharmaTruth but need to remain anonymous for business and personal reasons. Could someone call me on my private cellphone 818-207-2288?'

"What do you think?" Max asked.

"Sounds like a Russian plot." Casey laughed. "Let's call them."

"What if it's someone who's trying to undermine PharmaTruth?" Max said.

"Good thinking. Let's run it by Dr. Barrett before we do anything."

Casey pulled his headset from his kinky, reddish-blond hair, and they hustled down the hall to Tom's office. They showed him the note.

"Interesting," Tom said. "Gotta be careful. Let me call this person on my supposedly secure line. Trouble is, most phones are traceable. But maybe I'm being paranoid."

He dialed the number and put the phone on speaker.

"This is Dr. Tom Barrett. You found our website and asked for a call. What can I do for you?"

"Thank you for returning my call," a woman said. "I'd like to meet someone from your organization, but over coffee or lunch. Is that possible?"

"It's possible, but what's the purpose?"

"I'd rather not talk by phone. That's why I want to meet. I can email the name and address of a coffee shop. Could someone meet me there?"

"I'll open up my schedule over the next three days, and I'll check our site." Tom was fascinated, but still wary. "Can you include a description of yourself, so I'll know who to look for?"

"Sure. Thanks for doing this. I'm very nervous, so I'll hang up now."

Tom turned to Max and Casey. "I would have invited you to come, but three on one isn't conducive to sharing information. If it's appropriate after our encounter, I'll suggest she meet you later. Maybe this is the project you've been hoping for. At any rate, it's fun to speculate on what she has in mind."

Tom sat at his desk after Max and Casey went back to their perches on the website. *What could this woman be about? She sounds legit but you never know.* Logging on to his email, Tom saw the message pop up.

"Thank you again for meeting me. There's a coffee shop in the South End called Coffee Obsession on Tremont Street. I can be there at 10AM. I'm in my late thirties, brunette and will wear a Burberry scarf. I googled you, so I will probably recognize you by your online photo."

It was set. Tom figured if she were being this cautious, he'd better use security backup.

"George, got a minute to come to my office? Got a question."

He strolled in a few minutes later, coffee cup in hand.

"You must have another clandestine meeting you want me to monitor."

"You're psychic. How'd you guess?"

"Well, I haven't been doin' much since our Garden meeting, so I figured my MO was in monitoring your secret meetings."

"How about background checks on board members? Seems a little sneaky. What do you think?"

"My preference would've been to do it *before* you got them on the board. It's a little late and not sure you and I should be investigating your board. That decision should come from your board chair if there's a question about who to be on guard with."

"Okay, let it go. For now, though, I'm meeting with a woman who responded to our website. She seems skittish but that may be an act. I'm seeing her tomorrow at ten at Coffee Obsession on Tremont. Can you slip in a little before that?"

"Sure. Anything special you want me to do?"

"Just watch. You won't be able to sit close enough to hear the conversation, but I'd be interested in your take on her body language."

"Why does she want to talk to you?"

"No idea."

After George left, Tom dug into his pile of papers from various websites and news feeds. He was consistently sickened by recurring reports of unscrupulous behavior in health care. A recent bulletin reported that a prominent cancer center in New York had made deals with a large New Jersey health care system of hospitals, allowing access to their pool of patients. This was followed by their investing in a data analytics company affiliated with the hospitals. This smelled like a conflict of interest to Tom, but he put it aside. This wasn't really part of PharmaTruth, and he needed to focus, not get carried away by jousting at too many windmills.

He waded through more website messages; one caught his full attention. "The cost of my arthritis meds is going through the roof. What can you do about that?"

Tom leaned out of his office and motioned to his volunteer coordinator.

"Hi Leila. I just read this message from a woman who says the cost of her arthritis meds is, as she puts it, 'going through the roof.' Has anyone followed up on that?"

"No, I thought you might want to call her yourself. You know about AH Pharmaceuticals, right?"

"I know there was a newspaper article recently. I'll review it before I call her. Thanks."

Leila left and Tom searched for the article. It described how two giant makers of adalimumab began raising the drug's price in synchrony, ten times since 2013. A year's treatment in 2018 was $63,363, "according to one analysis." This represents an "almost 140 percent increase." The article went on to describe "extraordinary tactics used to preserve exclusivity of these drugs in the United States," despite much cheaper bio-similar drugs being manufactured in other countries and sold in European and other world markets.

Tom became more outraged as he read. Enormous profits were being hauled in by these two companies: in 2017, $18.4 billion and $8 billion respectively. Those two drug houses had increases in their profit margins of 36% and 43% in 2016. These price hikes were a serious threat to patients' health, despite vigorous denials by the companies. He rustled through papers and found the woman's name and number: Hannah Dorst.

"Hello," said a woman.

"Hi, this is Tom Barrett from PharmaTruth. I'm calling in response to your message posted on our website."

"Oh, thanks for getting back. Frankly, I doubted I'd hear from anyone. I've sorta given up on getting help. My doctors are fed up hearing from me, druggists too, and my friends are really sick of my bellyaching. But I'm in such pain all the time, I can't just do nothing." Tom could tell she was crying. "When I saw your website, I called. I'm not sure what you can do for me, but I'm at my wit's end."

"I'm not sure I can do anything for your pain, but I'd like to learn more about your experiences. I hope our organization can make changes in a system that isn't doing its job. Here's an idea. May I send a couple of medical students to listen to your story? They report directly to me, and we can take it from there. Okay?"

"When would they come?"

"I'll have them call. Their names are Max and Casey. You'll like them; they're idealistic young guys who want to change the world. I'll tell them as soon as we finish this call."

"I'll be glad to hear from them. Thank you for calling me back."

Tom hurried out to the message room, tapped Max and Casey and told them what he offered Hannah Dorst. They grinned, glad they had something concrete to do. Within an hour they had arranged to meet her.

***

Not much had changed in the South End since Tom's days at Boston Medical Center. The old brick bowfront, three-storied buildings on Mass Avenue, now apartments or condos, were once homes for the well-to-do of Boston. They were still handsome structures after years of wear and tear. He walked onto a side street where Coffee Obsession was crammed in between a barbershop and a convenience store. The scent of dark-roast coffee drifted out the door. Tom spotted a woman he believed was the one he was there to meet. Their eyes locked, and Tom moved quietly next to her and whispered, "I'm Tom Barrett."

"I'm Dina Robbins. Let's get our coffee and go over to that corner where we can talk." She nodded toward an isolated table.

Tom saw George sidle into a booth nearby.

"Never been to this coffee shop. Probably wasn't here when I trained at Boston Medical. Know when it opened?" Tom asked to start the conversation.

"No, but I've come here for about four years. Good coffee and sort of funky, with all the old broken-down couches and chairs. The wall library over there has old, yellowed books on almost everything."

Tom liked her immediately. She was open, friendly, and had an upbeat attitude. What did she want from him, from PharmaTruth?

"So, what can I do for you?"

"Let me tell you a little bit about myself. I'm a nurse/pharmacologist, now working for Pylea, a drug company in Cambridge. I became interested because Pylea took on a new drug for resistant post-op infections. My mother died due to renal failure after an MRSA infection not long ago, so I have a personal interest in seeing this drug succeed."

Tom's eyes widened when he heard this.

"Is this the drug that Ahmed Mohammed discovered?"

"Yes, how'd you know that?"

"I've known Ahmed for a while, in a different context. He's a wonderful human being."

"Yes, I've heard that. I want to meet him." She paused. "Anyway, I've been working at this place for a few months and have become, what should I say, disenchanted with the owner and the direction he's taking the company. When I saw your website, I thought I should talk to you. Confidentially, of course."

"You have my word on that. When you say, 'the direction he's taking the company,' what do you mean?"

"He wants to price this drug, which is cheap as hell to make, in the stratosphere, to make a pot of money for himself. I find this strategy unethical, even immoral, and I can't sit idly by and let it go. My mother suffered terribly, and I don't want to see others go through that when a drug is available and should be affordable."

"I see. Ahmed would be appalled if he knew this; he's a straight arrow." Tom glanced over at George, wondered if he should introduce him to Dina, but decided to wait.

"I'm sitting here, wondering how I can help. Have any ideas?" Tom said.

"I'm thinking of making notes of what's going on in meetings and in my interactions with the boss. He tells me a lot of things, insider information that I think at some point, if they persist on this course of action, must violate some statute, or at least if made public, would be bad publicity. Maybe a class action suit could be brought against them and information about their discussions and decision-making processes could be critical in court actions."

"Very gutsy of you. And dangerous. Are you aware of the risks you're taking if they found out?"

"Oh, they'd fire me for sure. But I'd have the conversations recorded, right?"

Time to bring George into their dialog. It might freak her out, but George could advise her about making secure recordings and how to stay safe personally.

"Right, you'd have the conversations, and that in itself is dangerous. You don't know what these people might do to get those and to keep you from disclosing what was said." He paused.

"Dina, I want to introduce you to someone I trust implicitly. I hope you aren't offended that I had him come here." Tom nodded to George, who rose and came to their table. "George Logan, meet Dina Robbins. George is a professional detective who works for our organization. I, too, must be vigilantly cautious because of this endeavor. He can counsel you about what you're planning."

George offered his hand to a surprised Dina, who rose from the table, took his hand and looked directly in his eyes.

"Um, th-this is a surprise. I don't know what to say. Frankly, I'm, well, sort of angry. It feels creepy to have been watched."

George looked at Tom, who looked away, worried that he'd blown this one.

"Tom's new at this, miss, so don't be upset with him," George said in his deep, most reassuring voice. "And frankly, everyone who contacts us through the website is a potential saboteur. I did overhear your idea about recording, and I'd like to tell you how to go about that. I want you to be safe while you do things that will get people very irritated. Tom and I have had some experience with that," he said with a wry smile.

Dina sat still, looking back and forth between Tom and George. Tom had the wisdom to keep his mouth shut while Dina processed what had just happened.

At length, Tom said, "I promised this would be confidential, and it is. Whatever transpires here, stays here. Even if you decide to walk out and do nothing more. But we're working toward the same goal, and we may be able to help each other. Want time to think about this, fine. Call me later if you need time to decide."

Dina breathed out a long sigh and shrugged.

"It was strange that you sprung George on me like that. But I guess I understand your needing to protect yourself." She smoothed her hair, pulled her collar up, tapped on the table with one finger, and looked at George. "Okay George, I'd appreciate your guidance on the logistics for making a safe record of what's happening and what's being said. And can we check in with each other?"

"Absolutely, Dina," George said. "Your safety, as well as the integrity of the intel you're providing, are my priorities."

***

The issues kept coming. Tom called Norman Wise to follow up on their discussion. He recalled an article he'd read about doctors paid to prescribe excessive opioids. It was another example of physicians being knowing accomplices to the escalating epidemic of drug addiction. The Massachusetts Attorney General had filed a recent lawsuit against a pharmaceutical company, saying it had "created the opioid epidemic and profited from it through a web of illegal deceit."

The company and their owners were in high dudgeon and denial. It would be years before the case would completely play out and even then, no matter who prevailed, the damage had been done to thousands of addicted patients. *How have physicians forgotten "primum non nocere-- first do no harm." How had morality gotten lost for them and the corporate executives who recruited their services?*

"Dr. Wise's answering service. How can we help you?"

Tom hung up. He didn't want to leave a message. He'd given Wise a secure phone to call but had not heard from him. How could he contact him without being discovered? Of course! George. He walked to George's office and found him staring at his computer. Tom explained the situation.

"Got his office address? I'll pay him a visit."

"Just walk in, no appointment?"

"I'll flash my private detective ID, the secretary'll let me by." George shook his head. "Tom, I'm a detective and this guy doesn't want to give away that he's changing teams. He's a professor, right? I'm in good shape. I'll put on a baseball cap to hide any grays, carry some old medical texts, and pop in on his office hours. I'm not even gonna talk about what you really want to know. I'll hand him a piece of paper saying he should call you, while I make up some BS about an independent study project."

Tom realized how little he knew about investigative work and was damned glad he'd met George at Zylinski.

"So, anything specific you want me to tell the good doctor?" George asked.

"I want to meet with him again, run some stuff by him. Set up a time and place for us. Thanks. By the way, how is the Security Unit coming along?"

"It's in hand. I've got some contract detectives on board for when we may need them. Things are picking up with Dina's involvement. My experience with this kind of work tells me there are times when things are seemingly slow and then BANG! All hell breaks loose. I'm preparing for that time, hoping it doesn't happen."

"I have a feeling you'll get busy soon, and then you'll be bitching about not enough time off." Tom laughed.

"So, you gonna get abducted again?" George teased.

"Oh God, I hope not. You're supposed to save me from that."

A few hours later, George called Tom; the meeting was set. Wise would meet him at Pho in Chinatown tomorrow at six.

Can I trust Wise? There's something odd about his coming forward to confess his sins, and to me, a guy he knows nothing about. And why am I having to pursue him? He kind of reminds me a little of Malcolm Crocker -- great bedside manner, then he gets those goons to beat me nearly to death.

Why am I thinking like this? Do my meds need to be adjusted? Are my instincts kicking in or is it in my head? My paranoia feels like it's creeping up to a higher level. Maybe I need to have Dr. Lyon check my blood levels. Probably time to reconnect with my buddies in my PTSD treatment group, find out how they're doing, if anyone's relapsed.

The next night he went to Chinatown around five to find Pho in a maze of narrow streets. Other restaurants that started in a similar basement den with two or three tables and take-out cubby holes had grown haphazardly into gaudy emporiums. Pho, one of the last authentic eateries, was deep down a backstreet in that miniscule island of little Asia. Tom found it after walking through throngs of chattering locals who jostled each other with abandon. Cigarette butts were strewn on the gutters and sidewalks, one of the few places in Boston to ignore warnings about smoking.

He ducked under an awning into Pho and found a table in an L-shaped alcove, out of sight of the front door. Just like in the movies. He ordered a pot of tea to wait for Norman Wise who poked his head in shortly before six o'clock. When Tom stood up to greet him, he noticed a Black man in a UPS hat and uniform taking a seat at the table nearest the door. George.

"Thanks for coming. I was getting concerned because you hadn't gotten back in touch," Tom said when Wise sat down.

"Sure, sure. Sorry. I've just been busy. How are things going on your end?"

Tom jumped into business right away. "Getting lots of hits on our website. One described some legal action against a company accusing them of inducing doctors to prescribe opioids. Know anything about that?"

"Oh sure, Purdue, everyone knows about that. And Insys, the makers of Fentanyl spray. Lots of wild parties and payoffs to prescribe various opioids. I'm one of the offenders, you know. Never got caught but another nail in my coffin of guilt. I'm glad it's come to light, but at the same time I'm scared I could get hurt. These things always get found out. Not that it will convince the denialists who don't want to believe. They pull their blanket of doubt over reliable data and decide that anyone with facts is a biased liberal."

"It's a discouraging time, but like most times. I'm trying to translate these revelations into solutions to effect change. Any advice?"

"Sure, sure, everyone is entitled to my opinion," he chuckled. "Seriously, though, I've thought a lot about it, and I believe we need legislation with big, sharp teeth to regulate the drug industry. These businesses represent capitalism gone berserk. They do whatever they damn well please, screw the consumer, the chronic loser."

As Wise talked more, Tom's trust in him grew. His initial skepticism was probably based on the curious way Wise came to him. His experience with Laxalta at Zylinski added coloration to his suspicions.

"In Europe there's much more regulation," Wise went on, "and their health care system works better, not perfectly, there's no perfect system, but better. Drugs are about a third cheaper on average, people have easier access, and their indices of health and well-being are better."

"So, what kind of strategy will get us from handwringing to action?"

"Advocacy in Congress," Wise said without hesitation. "Problem is, legislators from both parties get campaign money from pharma, and to make matters worse, they're utterly disconnected from real people's needs for health care. Lawmakers' own health insurance is like a Rolls Royce, and if they serve even a single two-year term, they get lifetime pensions and health care! What you need to do is find a legislator, if you can, who's got a family member without decent insurance experiencing a devastating medical problem. Remember, it was FDR who started the

March of Dimes, Kennedy's sister Eunice started the Special Olympics, and Bob Dole got the Americans with Disabilities Act enacted. That's what it takes."

"I have board members from different states. Maybe they can ferret out a couple of lawmakers who could be recruited."

"It would also help to have an insider, someone who has enough balls to blow a whistle. Takes a lot to do that. Whistleblowers almost always get punished for their good deeds."

Dina. What was her last name? He was glad George and Dina had met, even though it was awkward. He wondered if they'd met again to hash out how she could record what was going down with Warner and his ilk at Pylea.

"You willing to talk about deals you've made with drug houses? We need concrete examples. When we find a Rep or Senator to write legislation and conduct hearings, we'll have to have facts."

"For some reason, unknown to God or man, I've kept a journal. I must've known that one day I'd want to cleanse myself. I have a detailed accounting of my actions."

"Thanks, Dr. Wise," Tom said. "It looks like several things are coming together. We have a chance to do some good here. Please be careful. I'd keep that journal in a safety deposit box if it's not already in one, and hide the key."

Chapter 15

Dr. Rebecca Abrams had helped Dina enormously while she coped with her grief and her fury boiling up about the tragedy of her mother's death. Now Dina wondered, *should I confide in her about recording evidence of corporate wrongdoing causing a totally different kind of stress? Don't I have a moral obligation, not only to my mother's memory, but to future patients to expose this travesty? Doesn't that override loyalty in dealing with Warner and his kind? Is this even a topic to discuss with a therapist whose job had been to give me support after my mother's death?*

As she entered Dr. Abrams' office, she was still unsure. In that quiet time one has before a therapy session begins, she fidgeted with strands of unruly hair, fingers pressing her temples to stop the throbbing.

"What's going on with you? It looks like something is nagging at you," Dr. Abrams said softly when Dina's session began.

Dina's decision to tell her about her new mission was made easier by Dr. Abrams' insightful question. It felt like she cared.

"Well, I knew you were an accomplished therapist but didn't know you read minds. Am I so obvious?" Dina said, wondering if this transparency would work to her disadvantage in ratting on her boss. "I do have a new issue to talk to you about." As she told her about Warner, how his unbridled greed could make this life-saving medicine unaffordable for many patients and her plan to expose him, she repeatedly brushed back her hair and fidgeted with her collar.

"What makes you most nervous?"

"Big risks, as you can imagine. Like the risk of being found out and getting fired before I accomplish anything. The risk of not being believed, not making any damned difference at all," Dina said. She looked up at Dr. Abrams' bookcase, trying to make sense to herself. "Sorta like that woman who testified in the Senate about a Supreme Court nominee's sexual advances. Her own integrity was called into question and ultimately destroyed in the minds of millions by the press coverage. Too many people didn't care what he did as an adolescent. They attributed it to 'boys will be boys' behavior; they believed *him* when he denied it. Politicians, those in power do what they always do, and he got confirmed anyway.

"Honestly, I'm also scared of physical harm. Too many whistleblowers have disappeared or suddenly 'die.' Reminds me of the woman named Silkwood, you know, who died in an unexplained auto crash. Little things like that," she said with a wry smile.

"How are you weighing these risks?"

"No real way, it's too abstract," Dina said, shaking her head. "But I have a feeling, deep inside, that what I'm doing is the right thing to do. And if I don't do it, people could suffer, even die. I'll suffer with them if I'm given this chance to change things and don't take it."

"When do you have to decide?"

"Now. If I'm going to collect evidence, it has to begin right away."

"You're not a professional spy, Dina. Are you sure you have the stomach for this? And how will you keep yourself safe?"

"Actually, I won't be in this alone."

"Oh? You have reinforcements?" Dr. Abrams said.

Dina paused. *Was that question asked in my best interests or to gain information? Why am I revealing every little detail? Dr. Abrams was a prescriber. What if she's involved with one of the companies PharmaTruth is investigating?*

"I… I mean that I have friends who will support me…if I get stressed out."

"Sounds like you've made up your mind."

"I don't know. Maybe. Maybe not. But you're going to have to listen to me worry about this for, I don't know, maybe a long time, maybe only a few weeks. You probably shouldn't write any of this down or you could be like Daniel Ellsberg's psychiatrist, remember that? It's the one thing in civics class that stuck in my mind."

"Psychotherapists all know that story. The upshot is we make cryptic notes, have strong locks on our file cabinets and computers, have secret storage areas," Abrams said with a grin. "Secret handshakes, too.

"See you next week. And Dina," Abrams said, placing her hands on Dina's shoulders, "Take care."

Dina got in her car, called George and arranged to meet him at Coffee Obsession.

"First thing," George told her over their steaming coffee, "you can't wear a wire. If you've watched spy movies you may think that's an option. What you can do is keep a journal. It can be used to refresh your recollections for testimony in court or legislative hearings. This form of recording is universally acceptable into evidence, and you can bring those notes to proceedings like that. You might have to hand a copy over to the questioners, but that's okay."

"Should I do this on my computer or write it out?"

"Either way, as long as it's secure. You could get a device with voice recognition, talk into it and then hide it someplace."

"Like where? A loose floorboard?" She laughed nervously.

"Think of a place bad guys would never consider. That's not easy, I know, since I've been one to overturn people's dwellings to recover things, and there ain't many places I don't look. But use your imagination, think like a burglar and put it someplace else."

Dina took a sip of coffee and stared out the window. George watched her eyes as they followed a cyclist in the street. He hadn't noticed a scar near her right eye when they'd met before.

"Mind if I ask how you got the scar?" he said, pointing to his own eye.

"Oh...a...it's from a long time ago. Why do you want to know?"

"My investigative DNA. I can't help it. I'm curious by nature and my job reinforces that. I notice stuff, like no wedding rings on attractive women, and it builds a picture." George also noticed that she felt uncomfortable and didn't answer his question.

"And what kind of picture are you getting of me?" Dina said.

"You're bright, good-looking, and willing to take risks. But I don't know why. I wonder about that. I admire it but

I'm curious as to what lies behind it." He took a sip of coffee. "Do you have family?"

"Interesting technique – mixing in compliments with your interrogation."

"Oh, sorry. Just making conversation," George said. He was out of practice in the flirting department.

"One teenage daughter. Divorced. Both of my parents have passed. My mother died recently of complications after a postop infection. Did you overhear that when I met with Tom? That's why I'm so upset with Warner at Pylea for jacking up the price of a new antibiotic for resistant infections. Plain old money lust, no moral sense whatsoever. Just greed," Dina said. Her face turned red, and fingers tightened around her cup.

"Sorry. Didn't mean to upset you. I get it," George said. "It helps me understand your motivation, gives me reason to trust you. Because of my line of work, I'm naturally curious about altruistic people. Tom's that way and the reason I like working with him. I find that getting to know my clients – even though you're not exactly a client – but getting to know who I'm working with, helps me do my job better. And my job is to watch out for you and any others who could have trouble because of their dedication to PharmaTruth's mission."

Dina's hands involuntarily brushed her hair back. With a furrowed brow, she said, "You're the second person today who has underscored how dangerous this may be. It's beginning to freak me out. I know what I'm doing is risky and it's crossed my mind that I might be upsetting the wrong people, but is it a given that I could be hurt or just a possibility?" Dina chewed on a nail, an old habit that she thought was past.

"Don't mean to alarm you, but PharmaTruth is playing a high stakes game. Anytime you start messing with jerks in suits pulling down zillions of dollars in salary and bonuses, the potential for trouble goes up. From what I've found out about your boss Warner, he's not a nice guy. You said I was the second person who'd warned you about your activities. Who was the first? And can we trust them?"

"Oh, my therapist. Probably. Hopefully. If you can't trust them, all is lost. So, you've been checking Warner out?"

"Oh yeah, part of the job. He has a well-known track record in the drug industry. Managed to get a huge severance from Drum Drugs in Texas. I'm always amazed how companies give big money to creeps when they terminate them. Drum tossed him out because they were embarrassed by a slew of things he did. Messed up a good situation. He was pulling in about $10 million a year in salary and stock. He got arrested once for assault and battery of a prostitute. The judge in the Texas court where it was brought was a drinkin' buddy of good ol' boy Reggie. He dismissed the case based on the woman's 'unreliability,' a common occurrence in that court. Guess he headed East because his love of bourbon, womanizing, cigarettes and wild parties was causing too many headaches out West."

"I'm beginning to get the picture. Yuck." Dina leaned in and spoke in nearly a whisper. "George, do you think I'm a dope for trying to bring this guy down?"

"You're no dope. I'm just injecting a little reality into what you're doing. You're also no Mata Hari and are a bit naïve about this stuff. I want you to be aware, that's all. My job is to make sure you're safe. I take that very seriously. Keep me informed about everything you do," George said.

She looked at George quizzically. "You're going to be my protector, and I don't know anything about you. Can you fill me in?"

George told Dina the broad outline of his friendship with Tom at Zylinski's PTSD treatment program. He didn't tell her about their joint effort to expose corporate sabotage by a drug company. He didn't tell her that Tom's paralytic arm resulted from thugs who nearly beat him to death.

"You met while you were both patients?"

"Yep, we're both survivors."

"Where did you grow up?"

"Alabama. The true Deep South. Daddy was minister in a little Black church, Mama did a lot of sewing for white folks. They made sure I got a good education. I got into state university and got a degree in Black History, a new major in those days. I wanted to go to grad school but there was no money. Daddy was diabetic and got real sick about that time and Mama got breast cancer. I had to take care of them. So, I took an exam for a job with the local police department. They needed a Black cop and had to give me a job. I worked my shifts and took care of Mama and Daddy after hours. They died within a week of one another. After they died, I joined the military, mainly to get veterans' benefits to go back for my master's degree. But after I went berserk over there, charged into a group of enemy combatants, they sent me home with the diagnosis of PTSD."

Dina listened, mesmerized by this story of loss and resilience.

"I can't imagine what your life must have been like in Alabama. And losing your parents and plunged into that horrendous war." She sighed. "You're in a dangerous line of work. Who worries about you? Do you have a wife or girlfriend, kids?"

"No wife, casual girlfriends. Nothing serious. I was in no shape for a relationship after the Middle East War. I'm in no hurry. Ms. Right comes along, I'd consider it. Like to have kids someday. And no need for anyone to worry about me. Don't mean to brag, but training and experience have made me good at what I do."

George stood up, reached in his pocket and pulled out a phone.

"Use this phone -- and only this phone -- to get me. My number is in its directory, and you can add Tom's, your daughter's, or other people for emergency purposes, but not many. Keep it in a safe place, not your purse. Okay?"

"Okay. Thanks, George. I'm glad you'll be looking out for me. Should we meet from time to time?"

"Whenever you want, but better to talk on the phone."

***

When Dina got to her office, her secretary told her Warner wanted to see her as soon as she got in. Her pulse rate went up and her face flushed.

"Did he say what he wanted? Should I bring anything with me?"

"No, he just said to tell you he wanted to see you."

Dina hurried down the hall to Warner's office, knocked and heard him say, "It's open, come in."

"What can I do for you?" Dina said instinctively, then realized it was a double entendre she hadn't intended.

"Probably a lot of wonderful things." He winked. "What are you doing for dinner tonight?"

Surprised and flustered that the relationship she hoped to exploit for information was at hand, she said, "Well, I had no plans."

"Great, go with me to Valerio's. Seven okay?"

"Y-yes, seven's okay. Where's Valerio's?"

"Oh, I'll take you there. Meet you at my car. Don't think it'd be smart if we're seen leaving together, you know how office gossip runs. I have a red Ferrari parked near the elevator, first floor. Meet me there."

"You'll bring me back to pick up my car?"

"Well, we'll worry about that later."

It's begun. I know the drill: he'll invite me to his place, start his seduction routine, and then what? I'll string him along. He's a disgusting man, how can I respond to him in a way he'll believe? Just his repulsive cigarette breath laced with bourbon is enough of a turnoff but add that to a domineering and egotistical nature. Everything about him is repulsive. In the back of her mind, George's report on Warner's assault tried to wave a red flag. She ignored it. *If I'm to get him to confide in me, she thought, I'll have to fake being interested. Hope it's worth it.*

As seven o'clock approached, Dina fidgeted with her nails and hair, glancing in her mirror to see if anxiety was evident in tension around her eyes. Satisfied that she looked as usual, she slipped the phone George had given her into a side pocket in her slacks, picked up her laptop case, and went to the elevator. Most everyone had left for the day, but her secretary was still at her desk. *She can't be that busy. I haven't given her anything to do. Should I say goodnight?* She stepped into the elevator and waved to her, got a smile and a wave back. *She seems her usual sunny self. Maybe she just isn't in a hurry to go home.*

Warner was sitting in his car when Dina approached. He didn't get out but motioned to her to get in the passenger side. She opened the door, got a whiff of cigarette smoke, and sank into the plush white leather seat.

"Hi. Nice car. What kind is it? I'm not a car person."

"Most girls aren't car people. It's a Ferrari. Drives like a dream. Got it for about 350 K. I hear they have a cheaper model, but I always want the top of the line, in everything, including women." He smiled at her, thinking he was flattering her with this gratuitous comment.

"It's a beautiful car, no doubt about it."

Warner backed out of his VIP parking space, flashed his parking card past the sensor to open the gate, and turned onto Mass Avenue. When they got to Valerio's, he rose from his seat stiffly with a low groan, stood for a minute getting his bearings and passed his keys off to a turbaned valet. Making no move to assist her, he waited for Dina to get out, then headed for the entrance to the restaurant, letting her follow behind. *A real gentleman.*

The hostess fawned over him as she led them to a private room. A white cloth adorned the table that already had an opened bottle of wine with a towel wound around its neck, resting in a canister. A waitress stood at the ready.

"I ordered chardonnay since most women prefer white. I don't drink wine. That's for you," he said. He asked for a double shot of Jack Daniels, neat, no ice. "I prefer a real drink. Always have, since I was ten."

Dina sat down, smoothed her jacket and studied the menu. When the server came, she ordered fettuccini with clam sauce. Warner ordered antipasto for the table and veal scaloppini as an entrée. He barked at the waitress to bring bread, grated Parmesan cheese, and olive oil.

"Don't know where they get these girls, worse every time. They're dumb as posts, always tell you their name. I don't give a shit what their names are, and they always say 'perfect' no matter what you order."

Dina looked at his snarling face and wondered what she should say to this grumpy old man. She smiled. "Have you ever waited tables?"

"Hell no; that's woman's work, unless you're a queer."

"Some of the best waiters in Europe are men, you know," Dina said, not wanting to get into a discussion about sexual orientation. "And they make little conversation. They just take your order and go. Maybe you'd like them better."

"That may be true," he said, relaxing a little. "I spent some time in Italy when I was younger. I liked the country but some of the people were suspicious. Never knew which ones were Mafia. I always felt they were gonna knock me over the head with a blackjack, take my money."

"Ever happen?"

"No, surprisingly. Guess they could see I'd knock the crap outta them if they tried anything."

"Tell me about yourself," Dina said, changing the subject.

Warner smiled, glad to talk about the person he loved the most.

"Like I told you, grew up in west Texas. Went to the best college in the state."

"Rice University?"

"What? No. West Texas A&M.

"You want to know what's made me able to achieve so much? How I can be the savviest shark in business waters? My old man was a rough sonnavabitch. He beat the shit outta me from when I was two until I got outta there," Warner said. He took a long drink of his whiskey, exhaling a large sigh followed by a burp.

"And I know I have a rep for not respecting women; I'm not oblivious," Warner continued. "That's from my childhood too. Ma was a pansy, wouldn't ever stand up for herself. He whacked her around all the time too. She knew he was beatin' me but was too scared for her own skin to do anything." Warner stopped talking, looking directly at Dina. "I don't know why I'm telling you this. Maybe 'cause I need to talk to someone. I still wake up from a nightmare, always the same, where I'm locked in a room with him and his razor strap. Just as he starts whippin' me, I wake up, sweating and shaking all over."

Dina looked at this flawed man and compassion for him arose unbidden. "That's a horrifying way to live and awful to be trapped in that nightmare. Do you have any brothers or sisters?" Dina asked.

"No, don't think my parents had sex after I was born."

"Are you married?"

"Widower. My wife Edith died about ten years ago, cerebral hemorrhage. I still miss her. I've lived alone since then. She took good care of me, but I don't really need anyone now. I like my freedom. Make enough money to get my needs met. Edith and I never had children. I would've been a rotten father anyway, since my father taught me all the wrong ways to deal with kids.

"Are you married? Children?" he asked.

"Divorced. One daughter, senior in high school. Good person."

"You don't look old enough to have a teenager. She as pretty as you?"

Dina didn't want him to know *anything* about her. She wished she hadn't even mentioned Debbie. Maybe she should tell him her daughter lived with her ex-husband. She just smiled and studied her nails.

They chatted as they finished their meals. Dina was surprised at the slivers of charm that escaped. Then Warner yelled for the waitress.

"Got any brandy?"

"Yes sir, did you have anything in mind?"

"Cognac."

He chugged the brandy. "Spend the night with me," he said abruptly.

"You move fast, Mr. Warner." This was not a seduction. It was a command performance from her boss.

"We barely know each other."

"Jump in my car; we'll be home in a jiffy, and we can have a good ol' time. And you can call me Reggie."

"Reggie, thank you for an excellent meal and a nice evening. I'm just not like that, even though I do like you," Dina lied. She hoped she sounded sincere enough to put him off without causing a scene. And oddly, it wasn't a complete lie. He wasn't *totally* repugnant, not when you saw the hurt little kid in him.

Warner interpreted the rejection as fuel for the chase. A mere postponement.

"Speaking of liking things, how're you liking work so far? We gettin' any closer to our big announcement?"

"I love my job. And I love being part of the development of this new drug. It's exciting to see it moving along so fast."

"Can't move fast enough for me. I see big profit ahead. I'm gonna raise the price again. Made a couple of deals this week with a couple of big insurance companies. They'll pay whatever I ask. Course they'll slap on a big co-payment for the consumer, so it won't come out of their own profit."

"What about people who can't afford it?"

"Frankly, my dear, I don't give a damn, as Rhett said. If they're poor, it's their own fault. The undeserving poor, I say. What's important is profit. Life's all about profit. The report card of life is how much money you have."

Dina held her tongue since she didn't want to talk about his disdain for people and his misplaced priorities.

"Which insurance companies are you talking to?" she asked innocently.

He named two of the largest insurers in the country.

"Wow! How'd you get them to do that?"

"Promised the CEO's a bunch of shares in Pylea. The stock's cheap now, but once we release the drug, the stock'll rise like a rocket. Then these guys will get rich along with me. You ought to buy some stock now, too."

"I didn't realize insurance companies could buy stock like that."

"Oh, the companies don't buy the stock. The execs tell their wives or kids to buy it."

"A man of vision, I bet you have a lot of shares, yourself."

"A potful. Controlling interest, of course. You can't believe how rich I'm gonna be. You're lucky I'm interested in you. We can have a lot of fun together."

"Houses in the Caribbean and things like that?" Dina said, sticking to script.

"Yeah, and lots of first-class trips to fantastic places. What do you want? Clothes, jewelry, cars? If you're with me, you could have whatever your heart desires. I think I might even give up my other girlfriends."

"You have others?" Dina feigned surprise and shock.

"Yeah, but none as intriguing as you."

"Why, you don't even know me, and I haven't said I'd become involved with you."

"You will when you realize what I'm offering. I don't need to know you any better. I can tell you're terrific. I've known many women and know what they're made of. Women are easy to figure out, you know. I can tell you're quality."

Boy, what he doesn't know about women. But his generosity was touching. C'mon, he's a selfish, mean, smelly man. Don't be a fool and get swept away by visions of turquoise water and vacations.

She'd gotten valuable information and could hardly wait to record their conversation. As she thought about this, though, she felt a shiver go through her. This is what George was talking about, what Dr. Abrams was warning her about. This guy was not only loathsomely mercenary. He was dangerous. No sympathy for anyone, and he'd slit your throat if you crossed him. She wondered if he'd ever killed anyone. She'd ask George about his background check.

"Dina, you look so serious," Warner said.

"Oh, sorry. Tired, I guess. Would you mind bringing me back to my car? I want to be at the office early."

"If I must. But I'm sure there will be other nights that will end up much more satisfying," he said and winked at her.

Dina could manage only the weakest of smiles.

Chapter 16

Max and Casey pulled up to the modest triple-decker in Casey's ridiculously painted 15-year-old VW beetle. Although Hannah Dorst expected a visit from medical students from PharmaTruth, when she peered through her sheer living room curtains, some doubt arose about these two young men, dressed in khakis and ski jackets. They ambled up to a bank of doorbells, leaving Casey's weird car with one front wheel on the curb, the others on the street.

Casey pushed the button with a tattered card reading, "Dorst" and waited.

Hannah asked through the intercom, "Who's there?"

Max, not knowing how well it worked, bellowed, "We're Casey and Max from PharmaTruth."

Hannah used her intercom to let them in and told them to come on in. She was able to maneuver her walker out into the hallway.

When they got to Hannah's door, they encountered a bent-over woman in her late sixties. Clinging to her walker, knobs on the joints of her fingers tightly wound into her palms, face permanently fixed in a mask of discomfort, she appeared ancient to them. She made a brave effort to smile a welcome.

"So nice of you to come see me," she said, motioning them into her apartment. Outside her back window, Max saw crumbling wooden porches barely hanging on the rear walls of other triple-deckers behind Hannah's house. Inside her cramped living room, small figurines adorned bookshelves and a worn overstuffed couch with matching chairs spoke of Hannah's marginal economic situation. Walmart-framed, wrinkled photographs of children and grandchildren sat on a black, dusty upright piano with yellowed keys.

"Do you play that piano?" Max asked with enthusiasm, after they sat down.

"I used to. But look at my hands. They don't work anymore," she said. "Can I give you something to drink? Coffee, tea, tonic?"

"Oh, no thanks, Mrs. Dorst. We're here to talk to you, mainly," Max said. "Do you live here alone?"

"Yes. I take care of myself, it's hard, but I simply can't stand the idea of leaving my home. Some girls come in to help with chores. My groceries get delivered. I get along pretty well," she smiled at them warmly.

"Before we talk, would you allow me to play your piano?" Max asked.

"Oh yes! I'd love that. It's probably way out of tune but help yourself. It'll be great to hear live music in my home."

Max played Clare de Lune. Then a little riff on Begin the Beguine.

"Oh, that's so wonderful. Come back anytime and play some more!" Hannah beamed.

"It's not so out of tune," Max said. He looked Hannah straight in her eyes and said, "I'll be glad to come back and play for you." He looked at Casey, whose right leg was jiggling, a sure sign of his need to get on with things.

"Maybe we ought to do what we came to do. We need to know what problems you've had with your medications."

"Well, I got rheumatoid arthritis. You may already know that by looking at me, bein' medical students and all, had it for years. Before my husband died, he helped me a lot. Lately it's gotten worse. I been taking a drug called Humira. It's advertised on TV, you know."

She told them in detail about how the medication got more and more expensive until she no longer could afford it.

"If you don't mind my asking, what do you live on, Mrs. Dorst?" Casey asked, shaking his head in dismay.

"I got no secrets, so, no, I don't mind. Both Henry, my late husband, and I were teachers. I have a little pension from that, but that's about it. My landlord's been good about not raising my rent, but it still eats up a lot of my budget. I don't know what I'm gonna do, to be honest." Tears filled her eyes.

Casey's face flushed with sympathy and anger, but he resisted his impulse to start flinging expletives around the room. He was easily moved to indignation by over-identifying with people he thought had been treated badly by society.

"What about family? Have any kids who might lend a hand?" Max asked.

"My two adult children – one lives in Nevada, has three kids, no extra money. Lives from hand to mouth. Wife's been sick, may have something to do with drugs, don't know. My daughter in Oneonta just got divorced so she can't help, got her own problems. There are friends from the parish, but they can only do so much. It's hard to ask for help, ya know? Guess I'm too proud, or I hear Mom's voice sayin', 'pull up your socks and get goin'.'"

"Would you be willing to tell your story to the papers?" Max said.

"Geez, I don't know. I could get into a jam by complaining. You can't fight City Hall; you ever hear that? The thing is, after newspapers tell your story, reporters go on to another one, forget about you, but the finger's been put on you."

"That's for sure," Casey said. "Reporters look for headline stories and often forget who's endured them. But they got their jobs to do, report current news, or as they always say, 'breaking news.' But if you guys goin' through stuff don't speak up, how's the world gonna find out about your problems?" Casey asked, trying to be reasonable while holding in his frustration at her situation.

Hannah Dorst looked at him blankly, bewildered by her dilemma but afraid of consequences no one could know. Max gently took her gnarled hands in his.

"We're hoping to get laws passed in Congress to help, but we need people like you willing to talk about your difficulties," he said, looking straight into her eyes. "Give yourself some time to think it over. When I come back to play your piano, you can tell me how you're feeling about it, okay?"

"Oh, do come back! I love visitors, especially good-lookin' young fellas who play my piano."

***

On the way back to the office, Casey was fuming. His anger seemed to increase in tandem with the speed he was driving.

"It's so unfair! That sweet lady. Breaks my heart."

Max was worried he'd crash into someone. A VW Beetle was not the kind of car you want to be in when that happens.

"I'm so pissed off at fucking drug companies," Casey said. "Are they so removed from real people they can't see the Hannah Dorsts of the world? What's wrong with them?"

He cut off a red pickup turning left. The driver of the pickup was a big hairy guy in work clothes, tattoos everywhere. Casey ignored his bird finger when the light changed. Old rule of Boston driving: never make eye contact.

"Case, could you slow down?" Max pleaded. "I agree with you, of course. They live in a cocoon of like-minded people who rationalize everything they do, based on their distorted reality. They get support and reinforcement from each other." He paused for a couple of beats. "Just like we starry–eyed idealists do," he said, realizing they were tapdancing on soapboxes. "But it pisses me off, too. That's why I run five miles a day and have a punching bag in my room. But we gotta figure out a way to support and encourage Hannah so she can let the world know how she's been screwed. She's right, you know, about the reporters flitting from story to story, but they have to."

"Think they're all that way?" Casey said.

"I know a couple who really care. I'll call them, see if we can get them interested. Maybe they'll come with us to see

Hannah next time, with her permission of course, and a promise they won't report unless she gives a green light.

"The other thing is, we gotta talk to Tom. Get his take on how to handle this."

A couple of hours later, sitting in Tom's office, Casey had calmed down. He was still jiggling his leg, but he was quiet, at least for him. Max was cool, but it was clear from the set of his jaw that he was ready to do battle for Hannah. He told Tom about their discussion with her, sat back, and waited for his advice.

"She's the canary in the mine," Tom said. "There're thousands of Hannahs out there with variations on that theme. Insurance companies are so cozy with the drug pushers they agree to pay whatever they want, then raise premiums to underwrite their highway robbery, or increase the co-pays and watch their stock quotes spike. Disgusting."

"What strategy can change that, is my question," Max said. "As long as money buys legislators, what chance do we have?"

"We have to publicize the dishonesty, the skullduggery, the corruption until the voters demand honest legislators with enough backbone to regulate this," Tom said. "It's really about changing the narrative of healthcare in general, not an easy thing to do. It's not only the drug houses, but also the entire health industry that's chaotic." He paused, ran his fingers through his hair. "Another windmill. I've got to stay on one issue at a time, but as a doctor, I see my profession crumbling around me."

"Maybe we should find some good reporters and convince Hannah to talk with them?" Max pressed on.

"Do you know any reporters who might give us a hand?" Tom asked.

"My sister works at one of the newspapers. I'll ask her."

"Do it. Would it help if I came with you the next time you see Hannah? Before you try to get her to talk to reporters?"

"Wow, that would help a lot. We're young and inexperienced in Hannah's eyes, I'm sure. You would bring gravitas."

Tom couldn't help laughing. *Well, I'll be damned. They view me as a senior citizen. They see me as I used to see faculty when I was a resident. Come to think of it, those faculty people weren't much older than I am now. Guess I need to acknowledge I'm getting old and crotchety.*

His mind wandered. *Was I supposed to call Cynthia? Damn, I am getting old when memory fails me like that. Was I going to arrange a weekend in the Bahamas, or was she?* As he was about to call Cyn, his phone rang.

"Tom Barrett here."

"This is Barry Ringer, from La Jolla. I'm a friend of Katharine Mott," a deep baritone voice quavered. "Kath's had a terrible accident. She was surfing and a big wave threw her against a rock jetty. She's got a head injury. She's in ICU at UC San Diego."

Chapter 17

Tom closed his eyes and moaned. His first thought was about Hunter and Jeff.

"Where are the boys?"

"They're with me. As you can imagine, they're devastated. I'm devastated," Barry said. "Don't know if she told you about me. We've been seeing each other for about a year."

"I don't know what to say," Tom mumbled, his mind flipping through images of Katharine, from Danny's photos to his mental clips of their recent dinner with Ben Higgins. "Any idea how it happened? Was she surfing alone?"

"Apparently, she went out after work by herself. The weather reports were showing dark clouds moving into La Jolla, predictions of a big storm coming in. I guess she thought she could catch a few waves before it hit," Barry said. "A fellow walking on the beach saw the whole thing. Said this enormous wave came out of nowhere, swept her up and flung her on the rocks. It's overwhelming, thinking how awful it must have been for her."

By reflex, Tom's brain clicked into its clinical box. "What does the CT scan show?"

"I don't know any test results. I'm not next of kin so I don't have any standing."

"What about her parents? Have they been informed?"

"They're on their way."

"How did you know to call me?" Tom asked, glad he called, but confused.

"Kath told me about your closeness to Danny and said if she ever had any trouble to call you, you'd know what to do."

I wish I knew what to do. What can I possibly do?

"I can come out there. I'm no magician, have no clinical connections at UC San Diego and can't reverse what's already happened. But I can be there for Hunter and Jeff -- and you. I'll ask around and see if I can come up with any medical connections. I appreciate your call. I'd hate to have found out weeks from now."

"I'll pick you up at San Diego Airport," Barry said. "Let me know when. I'll bring the boys depending on how they're doing. Oh, text me a picture of yourself, and I'll do the same so we can find each other."

Tom put his head in his hands, recalling his high school Shakespeare class: "The world is out of joint, oh wretched spite that ever I was born to set it right." As he sank into melancholia, memories of Danny stood out in brilliant relief, stoking the embers of his post-traumatic stress. *Should I call Dr. Lyon?* Instead, he combatted his surging black mood by moving, physically and mentally. Rather than making reservations for a freeing vacation, he booked tickets for this unexpected and wholly unwelcome trip. Keeping busy was an antidote to grief.

How would Hunter and Jeff absorb this? Barry Ringer? No, she didn't tell me about you. Is he or someone else available who could be the kids' guardians if she died? The last time he saw Katharine he'd scuttled fantasies about a romantic relationship with her and Cynthia was large in his life. Now he was sorry but selfishly glad he'd not gotten more involved, even fallen in love with her. It would've been easy to do.

Danny and Katharine. A couple he hardly knew but so dear to him. One gone and the other suspended in an unknown and precarious realm.

"Hi Cyn, Tom here. Got some bad news just now. Actually, appalling news." He told her that Danny Mott's widow had a surfing accident and was in intensive care in San Diego. He needed to go there, see what he could do. He told her about Hunter and Jeff, her two children.

"I feel obliged to help. Danny was my best friend."

"God, those poor kids. Who'll take care of them while she recovers?" Cynthia said.

"I'll find out. And recovery is only one option, certainly the one I pray for. I don't know how serious this is. I don't know what to expect. I'm sorry about our Bahamas trip. We can do it later."

"Would you like me to come with you?"

"I hadn't thought of that. You want to come? Not a pleasant trip."

"This won't be easy for you alone. I'd like to help."

"I wonder if there'll ever be a time when being with me won't be an assignment to support me," Tom said, regretting it immediately. "Sorry, I do appreciate your offer. You're right. It won't be easy for me. It sounds bad. Can you get away for this, like tomorrow?"

"No problem. I'd already cleared my calendar for a possible trip to the Bahamas."

***

Cynthia looked out her window as their plane made its final descent into the San Diego airport.

"Jesus, Tom, we're going to run into those buildings!" she cried.

"Don't worry, Cyn. Every time I land here, I think that. But it's their usual descent pattern. Look, you can almost see what's on those computer screens in offices."

After collecting their luggage, Tom spied Barry Ringer, looking like the picture he'd texted: black curly hair touching his broad shoulders, about six feet tall, slender; someone who'd probably spent many hours with Katharine in her favorite sport of surfing.

"Hi Barry, I'm Tom; this is Cynthia," Tom said. Feeling a need to explain who she was and why she was there, he added, "Cynthia was head nurse in the Emergency Department at Boston Medical Center when we worked there."

"Nice to meet you," Barry said, shaking hands. "Wish there were a different reason. Thanks for coming."

"How's Katharine?" Tom asked.

"Not doing well, I'm afraid, but you should talk to the doctors. You'll understand things I don't, and maybe you can explain them to me."

Being back in an intensive care unit evoked familiar memories and made Tom envious of the staff as they went about their tasks. Tom and Cynthia headed for the nurses' station with Barry.

"These are the folks I mentioned," Barry said to a nurse. "Friends of Katharine who just arrived from Boston to see her. Dr. Tom Barrett's a surgeon and Cynthia's a nurse."

They went directly to Katharine's bed. Tom took one look and suppressed a groan. His eyes blurred as he saw a battered face, swollen with bruises and abrasions, a tracheostomy tube in her neck, and all kinds of monitors and tubing snaking around her body. Cynthia, who never had known or seen Katharine before, stood immobilized. A nurse with experience in seeing such cases, she felt the impact of this woman's plight in a different way. Her nurse's detachment didn't apply as tears coursed down her cheeks. She turned to Tom, slipped her arm around his waist. His good arm wound around her.

"How long has she been this way?" Tom asked, exchanging a glance with Cynthia, whose eyes locked on Tom's.

"Since she came in, a couple of days," Barry said, sadness in his voice.

Two doctors stopped at the nurses' station and talked to the nurse who nodded toward Tom, Cynthia, and Barry. Tom wondered if she had told them that a surgeon and nurse were visiting their patient. They came to the bedside and introduced themselves.

"Can you give me a sense of what's going on?" Tom said.

"Are you related to Katharine?" Dr. Blank, the ICU specialist, asked.

Tom briefly explained his relationship to Katharine and her family.

"I understand you're a surgeon. Heard the history?" Dr. Blank asked.

"Better start with that. I know broad outlines, but not many facts."

"A man on the beach saw what happened and called 911. He said she was surfing when a huge wave came and dashed her against rocks. Brought here unconscious, and she's remained so. Her initial CT scan showed an epidural hematoma, a parietal skull fracture, and early cerebral edema. We evacuated about 35 cc's of fresh epidural blood through a cranial incision when she first got here. We're hoping her brain swelling will subside. Usual treatment for cerebral edema, which, as I'm sure you know, is suboptimal. No other significant injuries."

"Thank you. Prognosis?" Tom, having been in coma from head trauma himself, harbored great hope she'd come out of this. An evacuated epidural had a better prognosis than some traumatic head injuries. Still, he hadn't seen the CT scans and didn't know how severe the brain swelling was.

"Prognosis? Well, Doctor, as you know, brain swelling's hard to treat, and the longer it lasts the worse the prognosis. If she comes out of coma soon, I'd be much happier. I could use the cliché that the prognosis is guarded but you know we really don't know. Sorry to be blunt, but that's what it is."

Tom and Cynthia looked at Katharine again when the doctors left.

"Anything you can tell me from your conversations with the doctors?" Barry asked.

"Not much you don't already know."

"Did they predict how long she's gonna be in a coma?"

"No way to know, Barry."

"What about how she's gonna be when she wakes up?"

"Also hard to say," Tom said. He didn't know much about Barry or his relationship with Katharine or Hunter and Jeff. Had their relationship turned serious since the last time he saw her? What did the boys think of him? He thought of Katharine's parents. He recalled Katharine speaking of them. They lived in Colorado, he recalled. Boulder?

"Do you know if her parents have come?"

"Yes, they're in a hotel in La Jolla. They've come to see her a lot. As you can imagine, they're very torn up. I guess they're late sixties, maybe early seventies. Seem with it and look fit. You wanna talk with them?"

"I suppose I should. They don't know me, might not even know how I fit into Katharine's life."

"I'll call them and see if we can swing by their hotel. They'd be glad to meet with you, I'm sure."

Tom looked at Cynthia, who'd been quiet since they left the ICU.

"How did you fit into her life?" she asked Tom, with no signs of jealousy, only curiosity.

"I wrote to her while I was in my PTSD treatment to tell her of my friendship with her husband and offered help if she needed anything. I visited her three times, here in La Jolla, met Hunter and Jeff on my first trip but haven't seen them since then. We can talk about it later," Tom murmured, conscious of Barry's presence.

"She was very fond of you," Barry suddenly said. "She spoke of you on several occasions. At first, I was jealous, you know, but she teased me out of that."

Barry went to get his car to go to the hotel. While they waited for him to pick them up at the hospital entrance, Tom told Cynthia more about his recent meeting with Katharine and Ben Higgins.

"I think that those meetings brought her closure about Danny's death. It was gratifying that I was able to help."

***

Barry drove them to the Colonial Hotel, and Katharine's parents welcomed them into their room.

"I'm Hunter. They call me Hunter Senior. This is Julie, Katharine's mother. Won't you sit down?" he said in a quiet monotone.

When Barry introduced Tom and Cynthia, a somber silence hung over them. Tom abhorred conversational vacuums and said, "First, let me say how deeply sorry I am about Katharine. Do you know how I knew your daughter?"

"I know you were with Danny in the war; she told me that," Hunter said. "She had high regard for you. She also told me you wrote helpful letters when she was at her lowest point. And that you came to see her a couple of times. Julie and I appreciate your caring enough to do those things."

"Can you tell us, as a doctor, how you think she's doing?" Julie asked.

"I'm not one of her doctors, so I should leave that to them," Tom said, evading a direct answer. "I can tell you that I was once in coma and here I am." He didn't want them to lose hope, so he excused himself from being a dark messenger. "Katharine's recovery will take time; I can personally attest to that."

The formidable question of young Hunter and Jeff hovered over them. Tom wondered who was taking care of them while they were sitting in this hotel, whether any discussions had been held about long-term plans. Maybe it was premature, but surely planning had to be considered. He hoped one of them would broach that subject.

"Who's caring for the children?" Cynthia said, surprising them with her candor.

"Their regular babysitter. Clearly that's not an arrangement for them if...," Barry said without finishing the thought on everyone's mind. "They're also going to need therapy and a lot of support."

"Glad you brought this up," Hunter said. "Katherine's brother's not available, we know that. Julie and I are not young, but we've got to do something. We're their grandparents, aren't we? Bringing them to Boulder to live with us might be an option, but we'd be pulling them away from their friends, the house they've always lived in. Barry's offered to help, but just how isn't clear to us or to him. So, we're thinking about it, hard."

Tom listened, nodding. *What's my responsibility?*

"I want you to know," Tom said, his eyes looking first at Hunter and Julie then resting on Barry, "that I'll do whatever I can to help. I'm not sure what that will turn out to be, but I'm only a phone call away."

"It's been good meeting you," Julie said. "And we will stay in touch. I pray for Katharine, but I know she's very sick. We'll figure this out somehow. Thanks for being here with us."

Tom saw where Katharine's strength had come from. In the morning, he and Cynthia checked with the nurses at the hospital before boarding their flight back to Boston. Not much had changed. Tom knew it would take time before they would know her outcome.

Once he and Cynthia were seated, he slipped his right hand into hers. She tilted her head onto his shoulder.

"What do you think?" she said.

"I wish I knew what to think. If I believed in a god, I'd say it's in His hands. I might even say a prayer."

Chapter 18

Dina got to work early. She wanted to arrive before Warner, to settle her nerves and experience some normalcy in her job before his inevitable beckon. She busied herself with the promotional campaign, her enthusiasm paling since she now saw it as a money grab for Pylea, not a breakthrough for patient care.

Warner showed up around ten, and as expected, called Dina a half hour later. As she approached his office, she saw Roy Shelby slipping out, heading down the hall in the opposite direction. She knocked and was told to come in.

"Good mornin' to you! Had a great time last night and want to schedule another," Warner announced.

"I had a good time, too," Dina managed to say. "I have plans with my daughter coming up, so I'll check my calendar."

"You do that. I enjoyed our date mightily. Now I need you to get your sweet behind to work and get our marketing strategy set. We're gonna release Cidal in the next couple of weeks. I want a big splash, lots of coverage from the media. Coordinate with Shelby, he's savvy about such things. Talk to you later."

"One thing I need to know: what's going to be the final price?"

"My insurance guys say we could go even higher than $500,000, but I'm sticking with $500,00 for the whole package. Signed, sealed, and delivered to hospitals. Shelby will tell you about a couple of infectious disease guys from two of the biggest hospitals in town, who're willing to say good things about this drug. We've paid them well for their endorsement."

"What were their prices?" she asked, knowing he'd confide in her.

"Cheap. Four weeks in Hawaii, all expenses paid, for their families."

More grist for the mill. Glad he didn't hesitate telling me.

"You mentioned Dr. Mohammed. I'd still like to meet him."

"I'll get him over here today. He'll come whenever I call him. He's like my lap dog," Warner said with a smirk.

Dina had seen small glimmers of redeeming qualities in Warner, but any liking of him was quickly melting away as he continued to display abominable behavior. At some level she still felt sorry for him. His childhood was a perfect recipe for making him into a sociopath, but that didn't excuse his immoral behavior, did it? She knew she had to contain her disgust for him while she got more incriminating evidence. She'd already recorded many of his statements, both in the Council meetings and last night when his tongue was liberated by alcohol. His recent boast that he'd bribed doctors to promote Cidal was gold. But she yearned for the day when this was history.

***

Ahmed Mohammed sat down in the conference room with Dina around two in the afternoon.

"I'm so glad to meet you, the man who discovered Cidal! What a sense of accomplishment you must have," she said, holding his handshake a moment longer than usual.

His dark complexion didn't display a blush, but Ahmed looked down in embarrassment. His innate modesty was often tested like this, but he'd never gotten used to it. A colleague told him that he shouldn't bow his head in humility, as was his natural response when he was complimented, but to hold his head high and smile.

"I'm part of a team, so we are all the discoverers, not me alone. I'm very glad to have been a participant and hope the medicine will help patients," he said. "Do you know when it will be available?"

"We're preparing an announcement soon. Is there anything you want us to say about it?"

"Only that we hope this drug is not necessary often. Good care in hospital settings should include the best possible conditions for germ-free surgery and after care. But if this medicine is needed, we hope it will be given quickly."

Not the kind of thing Warner would want us to say. He'd say every postop patient should have Cidal prophylactically to prevent all potential infections. Dina the pharmacologist knew the surest way to make the drug ineffective down the line would be that kind of overuse, encouraging emergence of more resistant organisms.

"We'll include your hopes in our presentations," Dina said, knowing this idea would be shot down by Warner. "Anything else?"

"We hope it will be priced low to make it accessible to all who need it."

Dina couldn't tell Ahmed the truth without revealing her true feelings and exposing herself as the mole she was.

She simply nodded her head and stared out the window. "I'll do my best to influence that," she said, considering her words carefully. She hoped that sometime in the future she'd have another opportunity to talk with Dr. Mohammed to tell him what Pylea was doing, but not today. She was not far enough along in her mission to take off her mask.

After meeting with Ahmed, Dina went into her office, closed the door, and recorded all she'd learned that day. Her entries were growing. She needed to get them to George before long. Just as she was finishing entries into her notebook her assistant opened the door. Startled, Dina dropped her notebook on the floor.

"Anything else you need? It's late and I need to leave," she said as she beat Dina to the notebook. Picking it up, she glanced at it before handing it to Dina.

"Thanks. See you tomorrow," Dina said, trying to be nonchalant about her notebook. *Could she have noticed the entries? And would she have any idea what else was in that notebook? My door was closed, and she barged right in. Got to be more careful.*

Chapter 19

Gwen Allen winced in pain as she leaned over to pull on her compression hose. Her doctor had suggested them to combat worsening discomfort in both legs. How could she, at age thirty-eight, have pain she thought was reserved for senior citizens? Her back hurt in practically all positions and the shooting pain down both legs brought her to the edge. She had to find out what was going on.

She'd tried remedies advertised on TV and in supermarket magazines promising a cure. None worked. She tried acupuncture, chiropractors, physical therapy, yoga, and special diets. She'd lost weight, did Tai Chi, and went swimming. When she called her doctor, he referred her to Dr. Wallach, a neurosurgeon, at Suffolk General Hospital. After his exam and imaging studies were complete, she sat in his consultation room as he told her his opinion.

"Your symptoms point to spinal stenosis and disc disease. The MRI confirms that. What kind of work do you do?"

"I'm an accountant."

"You sit most of your day?"

"Yes, but I work out three times a week," she said defensively. "What's spinal stenosis? Never heard of it."

He explained it was narrowing of the openings between the blocks of bone in the spinal column that allow nerves to leave the spinal cord and carry messages to and from distant muscles and skin. He laid out several options for treating it, including an operation.

"A laminectomy is a surgical procedure that makes more space for these pinched nerves. It's successful in most cases, and I think you'd benefit from it. You'll get pain relief, and your life will be a whole lot better." He conveyed obligatory cautions, possible complications, and what she could expect postoperatively. She told the surgeon she'd think about it. The prospect of an operation on her back was terrifying. She'd heard plenty of stories about complications from back surgery. But she hoped not all back surgery was the same.

She couldn't sleep, not only from sciatic pain traveling down her legs, but also from the dread of going under the knife. She's lost both parents after cancer operations. *But those had to be different. They had life-threatening diseases and surgery couldn't cure them. But I can't go on with this pain. I must do something.* The next morning, she called Dr. Wallach's office.

"Please tell Dr. Wallach, I'm ready to go ahead with the, uh, lamectomy? What do I need to do?" she asked Penny, his office administrator.

"Laminectomy," Penny said. "We'll schedule a time and get back to you with pre-op instructions, okay?"

***

Gwen groped her way out of post-anesthesia haze and felt no pain in her legs or back. Was this relief from surgery? Already?

The nurse told her part of her relief was pain medication but that most patients felt better after this procedure. Two days later she was discharged with pages of instructions about postop activity and a prescription for one hundred OxyContin tablets. She was able to walk without pain, but the nurses insisted she get into a wheelchair to catch her ride home to Southie.

Her hospital social worker had already arranged for home health aides to come to her home since she lived alone. But she felt she could cope, because for the first time in many months, she had no sciatic pain, only lingering postoperative pain in her back, relieved by the Oxycontin tablets she took religiously. They made her feel peculiar, with nightmares and weird thoughts, but the doctors told her to take them.

By week's end she felt well enough to go back to work. She continued to take the opioid tablets. The doctor must have expected her to finish taking all one hundred pills in the prescription, part of routine postop rehabilitation, she figured.

Two days after her last dose, Gwen woke up from a nightmare feeling jittery. She threw off her covers and hurried to the bathroom. Looking back from her mirror was a woman with fright jumping out of widened eyes. Her hand shook reaching for a toothbrush. In a frenzy, she brushed her teeth and scurried back to the bedroom, confused by what possessed her body. Drops of mucus fell from her nose, muscles cramped as she paced. She peered outside, desperately hoping light would tame the glittering images in her head.

Iris, Gwen's home health aide, promised her she'd check in with her after her last visit two weeks before. Standing at

Gwen's front door, Iris knocked several times before Gwen heard her, so preoccupied was she with her strange mental state. Becoming aware of pounding noises, she rushed to the door and flung it open. She hugged a startled Iris, pulling her in.

"I'm feeling crazy," she told her with tears coursing down her face. Iris quickly looked at her and understood.

"You takin' your pain meds?" she asked.

"No, I finished them a couple of days ago. Why?"

"What were you takin'?"

Gwen ran to her medicine cabinet and showed her the empty bottle.

"What I thought," Iris said. "You be havin' drug withdrawal."

"What should I do?"

"Git your duds on. We're goin' to the emergency room. You need some help."

By the time they arrived at the ER, Gwen had chills and nausea. Her blood pressure was 190/120, so high they started an IV in case they needed medicines in a hurry. Iris explained what was going on. The nurse sighed.

"It seems that's all we do these days. Take care of opioid addicted people."

"Addicted? What do you mean?" Gwen cried.

"You taking opioids?"

"Yeah, I had back surgery and they gave me a prescription."

"How many did you get?"

"A hundred."

The nurse rolled her eyes, and said, "What kind of surgery did you have?"

"Lamectomy."

"Laminectomy. That doesn't usually cause a great deal of pain, so why'd they give you so many?"

"How should I know? I just did what the doctor told me to do," Gwen said in exasperation.

When the ER doctor was told the story, he came in and told Gwen he was referring her to an addiction clinic for advice and treatment. "In the meantime, I'll give you a script for a few opioid pills until the clinic gets you on Medical Assisted Treatment."

"Everyone keeps calling me an addict. I've never been addicted to anything. Never smoked marijuana, never took cocaine, nothing. I don't even drink alcohol. How can I be called an addict?"

"Unfortunately, you're called an addict because you're addicted to opioids. Not your fault, but there you are. But the clinic can help you. Get this prescription filled to relieve your withdrawal symptoms, then go to that clinic. Go soon, because this script is for just ten pills. And it's non-refillable. I don't want to be part of your problem."

Gwen held the script in her shaking hand, hoped it would dampen her jitters and aches.

"Iris, please stand with me in line," Gwen said as she swayed back and forth at the drugstore, trying to offset pains in her shoulders and neck. "You know how to get to that clinic?"

"GPS will get us there. We should go there right after this."

A woman strolled behind the pharmacy counter and narrowed her eyes as she looked at Gwen when she handed her prescription over. Gwen felt blood rise in her face. *She's judging me, she thought, and assigning me to that same pigeonhole reserved for scruffy bums who shoot up in alleys.*

Humiliating. Degrading. How did I get to this place? She was ashamed now that she used to have so little sympathy for druggies, as she called them, how she thought they all deserved to be in jail. Now she was an addict. *Unbelievable.*

When Iris and Gwen found the clinic, they were greeted by a friendly young woman and were seen within minutes. Gwen told her story, and a nurse nodded in understanding.

"We'll start you on MAT, short for Medical Assisted Treatment. It substitutes a different, less addictive drug, for opioids. It works for a lot of people."

"I just got a small prescription filled for more opioids. Should I take any of that?"

"Not after we get you started on MAT."

Now I have to take another drug because some hare-brained doctor put me on an unnecessary and addicting drug. Her heart rate accelerated, and her face flushed with anger. *I want to get even with that jerk for prescribing this. But how? A lawyer? Costs too much and takes forever. Maybe on the web I can find some way to go about getting some satisfaction for the wrong that's been done to me.*

Gwen spent a lot of time on Facebook, Twitter, and surfing. She searched "opioid addiction," and hundreds of sites came up. Clearly, this was a big deal affecting lots of people. She narrowed her search and read through home pages for dozens of websites, but none satisfied her. Just as she tired of searching and was about to stop, she came upon a website called PharmaTruth. One line stood out:

"Addicted to opiates because a doctor over prescribed opioids"

She called the number.

***

After screening calls on PharmaTruth, Leila took a stack of messages to Tom. He knew Gwen's addiction to opioids was a sentinel case for charges he would bring against offending drug companies. In 2007, according to court documents, AH Pharmaceuticals, which made the opioid tablets, was fined $600 million in federal court for "fraudulently marketing opioids." Despite this, since that fine was paid, a suit by the Attorney General in Massachusetts stated that the company had sold more than 70 million doses of opioids in Massachusetts alone, for more than 500 million dollars.

"Is this Gwen Allen?" Tom asked when a woman answered.

"Yes, who's this?"

"Tom Barrett from PharmaTruth. I'm calling in response to your message on our website. I'd like to talk to you more about your case. Is that possible?"

"Oh, goodness, thank you so much for calling. I didn't expect to hear anything, you know, you seldom do. I'd be happy to talk with you. How can we do that? Over the phone? In person?"

"I can come to your home, or you can come here, whichever is easiest for you."

"I'm just beginning my MAT so if you could come here that would be appreciated."

"I'll ask my secretary to set up a time and get directions. See you soon."

Chapter 20

George noodled around on his computer as his mind wandered. *How does Tom plan to turn his idealism into action?* Meetings with Dr. Wise and Dina were eye-openers about deep veins of corruption running in the mines of Big Pharma. George heard a lot of Tom's talk about dual legal and legislative pathways to expose and change the mountains of unethical, borderline illegal and clearly criminal behaviors.

The aching frustration for George was fueled by known realities: lawyers are platinum-plated, legal settlements take forever, and hearings in legislatures move slower than traffic on the Southeast Expressway at rush hour. But at least hearings were public. They made news and might compel CEOs to leave their cocoons of executive suites and sweat in front of cameras while grilling by lawmakers exposes their vulnerabilities. Constituents want relief from burdensome drug prices now. Pressure was building for Congress to get something, anything, done.

Tip O'Neill famously said, "All politics is local," George recalled. Who's the more likely of senators from Massachusetts to take interest in this?

He searched the Senate membership list and found Senator Sean Rafferty's website. His record in the Senate was moderate, sort of center-left, and he'd sponsored some legislation about Medicaid expansion. George knew low-level assistants screened messages on websites, so he used his phone instead. At least you could negotiate with assistants by phone, and if necessary, bully your way to contact with the Great Man.

"Senator Rafferty's office, Laney speaking. How may I help you?" a well-polished voice said.

"My name is George Logan, one of Senator Rafferty's constituents. I want an appointment to see the senator to talk to him about abuses in the pharmaceutical industry."

A long pause.

"Are you there?" George said.

"Uh, oh, sorry, yes, I'm here, trying to jot down what you said. Senator Rafferty will be in the Commonwealth next week, but he's booked solid. Can I put you on an on-call waiting list?"

"No, that's too uncertain. I'm an investigator with a non-profit company called PharmaTruth. I have information about the pharmaceutical industry the senator needs to know about."

Another pause, a shuffle of papers.

"I'm looking for possible openings." After another interval, she finally said, "I can squeeze you in early morning, next Tuesday, say about 8:30 AM. Can you make that?"

"Yes. Where?"

"You know where the JFK Federal Building is?"

"Our office is on Beacon Hill, so, yeah, I know. Thanks."

George mused about what Jack Kennedy would have thought about the building bearing his name. The JFK Federal Building had no unique architectural features distinguishing it from hundreds of other modern urban buildings. It seemed a shame that in Boston, where so many significant historical structures graced the city, this mundane edifice would be named after an erudite president who appreciated antique edifices.

He was shown into a small conference room, and within a few minutes, surprisingly, Senator Rafferty stepped in. A tall, slender man with swept back white hair and a narrow face, fixed his piercing blue eyes on George, who rose to greet him.

"Good morning. Have we met before?" Senator Rafferty said.

"Never had the pleasure. Good to meet you," George said.

"Please, please take a seat," he said. "You want to talk about pharmaceutical companies, right?"

"Yes. I'm an investigator working for a non-profit called PharmaTruth." George handed him his card. "Briefly, our mission is to call attention to questionable practices of pharmaceutical companies. I know you've sponsored important legislation on Medicaid expansion and that's the reason I felt you'd be interested in our mission."

"A timely topic, one I *am* interested in. Pharmaceuticals have been going unchecked, far as I can tell. What's your outfit actually doing?"

"Developing strategies to combat the runaway greed of big pharma. One tactic is to gather stories from real people about how they've been screwed by drug manufacturers. Putting a human face on what's happening."

"How are you going to use those vignettes?" Rafferty asked. George could see why this guy kept getting re-elected. He gets it without a lot of discussion.

"We're recruiting news media to get the word out about these practices. I'm here to persuade you and other legislators to conduct Congressional hearings where company honchos are under oath to provide inside information. Legislation coming out of those hearings could put serious brakes on their misbehavior," George said. "And, I might add, give political capital to you guys in white hats for the next election."

Rafferty, used to constituents' awe in his presence, sat surprised, hearing George's action plan presented with such certainty and confidence. Diplomatic by nature, he needed time to collect his thoughts for a response. He stared at George, who returned his gaze without flinching.

"Well, an ambitious project," he said. "I need to ponder how to operationalize all you've said. I'm close to the Chair of the Senate Finance Committee where hearings like this might take place. We'd need similar House hearings, probably from the House Oversight Committee. I know the Chair over there, too. Let me think this through and get back to you, okay?"

"I appreciate your interest, Senator. My boss, Dr. Tom Barrett, would welcome your visiting, to meet our staff and Board of Directors. I think you'd be impressed with the caliber of people involved."

"I'd like to send my chief of staff to your office. Would that be of interest?"

"As a first step, yes; but after that, we'd like *you* to come." George knew he was overstepping, extending an invitation to a U.S. Senator without Tom's knowledge, but he thought he'd get away with it, especially if it came to pass. "When can I expect to hear from you?" he said.

"Soon," Rafferty said, seeing a persistent advocate across his desk. "I can see you won't let me tarry very long." He smiled.

George thought he detected respect. *Not bad between a Black ex-cop and a white senator.*

Chapter 21

"Where do we stand on contacting insulin-dependent diabetics who've responded to our website?" Tom asked Leila.

"We've gotten back to most of them to ask who'd tell us their story."

"As I recall we have several willing to do that, right?" Tom said as he perused the list on his computer.

"We have several, yes. We need to find the best ones to help us."

"Leila, did you know there are over 30 million diabetics in the States and about 7 million take insulin?" Leila nodded, knowing Tom was about to say more. "Looking over this list it seems that this woman Barbara Simon would be the best candidate to bear witness, keeping all the others on tap to re-enforce the argument."

Barbara Simon, a thirty-year-old woman, was emphatic when she'd responded on the website. She was articulate when she told of her alarm about the constantly increasing cost of her insulin. She lived in Brookline, a plus since Max and Casey could easily visit her.

"Casey, Barbara Simon is a type one diabetic, has taken insulin since she was ten years old," Tom said. "Get in touch with her. She works days, so call after seven PM. If you can visit her, find out if she'd be will also to talk to a reporter. Has Max gotten a name of a trusted reporter yet?"

"I'll ask. I'll call Barbara Simon tonight. Know anything else about her?"

"No, that's for you to find out. You guys are skilled at mining information from people. You'll be good doctors since you take good histories." Casey smiled with satisfaction at the compliment.

When Casey called Barbara Simon, her husband answered after the second ring, letting him know she wasn't available.

"Well, my name is Casey Andrews and I'm calling from PharmaTruth. Ms. Simon left a message on our website to call. Can you please give her a message to call me?"

"Yes, I'll tell her. I think I know what this is about. She'll be back from an errand soon. What's your number?"

About a half hour later Barbara Simon called.

"I posted on your website because my insulin keeps getting more and more expensive. I have insurance but my monthly out-of-pocket cost is close to $900.00. I was hoping your organization could do something about this."

"I work with another medical student for PharmaTruth, and we're collecting stories of people who're having difficulty paying for their medicine. Is there a time we could come see you at your home and get more information?"

Several nights later, Casey and Max found Simon's small Victorian house on a side street. They rang the bell and waited.

"Hello, you must be from PharmaTruth, right?" a slightly overweight, blonde woman said. She opened the door with a smile.

"I'm Casey, this is Max."

"Come in, this is my husband Charles and my son Mark. He's four."

Mark looked at them suspiciously, then turned around and scampered into a small room where a television set was flickering. Charles shook hands with them and showed them into a room with a small bay window looking out to the street. A few hooked rugs were scattered on the shiny hardwood floors. Max and Casey sat in straight-back Shaker chairs and the Simons sat on a love seat opposite them.

"Thank you so much for allowing us to come to your home," Max said.

They listened attentively as he told them PharmaTruth's mission.

"Could we have your permission to record this conversation?" Casey asked.

"Of course," they said in unison, without hesitation.

Casey prepared his iPad, while Max began the interview.

"What we're hoping to do, Ms. Simon, is to hear your medical history and some specifics about how insulin prices have changed since your diabetes was first diagnosed. We hope to put it together with other personal stories about drug costs and publicize them in the media. Ultimately, we aim to present these at hearings before congressional committees who will consider proposed legislation to lower these excessive costs."

Barbara gave them details about her private medical information, surprising in its candor and transparency. She had tracked the cost of her insulin making it apparent that the cost has risen nearly 1000 percent since she began treatment as a ten-year-old child.

"As I said, we have good insurance; we can afford the $900 per month out of pocket, although it certainly impacts our finances," Ms. Simon said. "Both my husband and I work, but many people, especially those with advanced cases of diabetes where they have numerous complications, can't afford to get the meds they need. I think that's criminal."

"Are you willing to go public with your story? Like, talking to a reporter, telling your story before congressional committees, maybe even testifying in court?" Max asked.

"Yes to all of that. I'm furious that we, as patients, are being held hostage because of our illnesses, not exactly our fault, you know? Anything I can do to change that, I'm all in."

"Thanks, Ms. Simon, for letting us collect this information, and we especially appreciate your willingness to share it with the general public," Max said. "We hope to bring about change because of people like you. We'll be back in touch soon." Max left one of his newly minted cards. "Call us if you think of anything else."

Chapter 22

The following morning, Tom riffled through messages on his desk. On top was one from Max about meeting with Hannah Dorst.

"Max, let's set a time for us to meet with Hannah," Tom texted.

In the taxi on the way to Hannah's Dorchester apartment, Tom asked Max if he'd spoken with his sister at the newspaper.

"Yeah, I have. She's gonna talk to the Searchlight Team to see if someone will join us when we see Hannah the next time, assuming she's willing to talk with a reporter."

"Great. Max, take the lead with Hannah. Casey, take some notes? I'll get involved when it seems appropriate."

Hannah watched them from her window. When she saw them getting out of the cab, she began her slow journey across the room. Her hip and knee joints sent painful signals as she hobbled to the buzzer to open the door. She greeted the threesome with a big smile.

"I have tea, coffee and some goodies. What would you like?" Hannah said, thrilled to have them in her living room again. After they introduced Tom, Max and Casey helped themselves to chocolate chip cookies and tea, then relaxed into their seats. Max knew what Hannah expected. He offered to play the piano.

"Wonderful! I have a request. Can you play Clair de Lune again?" Hannah said.

Max smelled the furniture polish Hannah had applied to the wrinkled finish of the ancient piano and noticed the major keys were several shades lighter than on his last visit. Hannah, with all her disabilities, had been working on this instrument, anticipating his next performance. Max barely suppressed a tear.

Tom was impressed with Max's finesse as his fingers skipped flawlessly over the keys.

"If you hadn't gone to medical school, you could've played at Carnegie," Tom said with a big smile.

Max threw up his hands in mock anger. "That's what I told Dad, but 'you must have a profession,' he said. 'A musician has no security.'"

Casey glanced over at Hannah and reminded everyone of their reason for this visit. "So, Hannah, how are you feeling?" he said.

"Not so well, sorry to complain. Ran out of medicine. My insurance company says my prior authorization has expired so they must process it again. That will take months."

"Do you have anyone to help with this situation?" Tom asked, seeing Hannah's fingers curled into a permanent fist. She was barely able to push her stiff, painful body up from the threadbare couch, a widow living alone.

"One of my friends, she's got arthritis too, tried to help, but she gave up, same as me. A social worker at the hospital offered to help but she works full time, so she's not available much."

"I heard about a service called Nurse Ambassadors, or something like that," Casey said. "Can you call them to help?"

"That's a joke, too. If your insurance doesn't cover them, they won't come. And I hear the real reason they come is to be sure patients continue getting prescriptions for the medicine their company makes."

"You must be pretty discouraged," Tom said. "I know we are, hearing this and other stories like it." He paused, trying to choose appropriate words to persuade rather than frighten Hannah. "One way to change how medicine gets to patients, regardless of their insurance coverage or ability to pay, is to get the word out to a lot of people about how unfair this system is. People are basically good, I think, and they also know that they might someday have similar problems."

"Yes, I do believe people care. There are some bad ones, but I agree that most people are good. But how're you going to get the word out?"

"One way is to get reporters from newspapers and TV to talk to people like you, write about it, and talk about it on TV." He stopped, letting the thought linger.

"Would you be willing to help by talking to a reporter?" he asked in a quiet voice.

Hannah stared at Tom, and he worried that meant "no." Hannah took a sip of tea, fumbled a cookie into her mouth, and looked back at him.

"Guess I'll talk to a reporter if it'll help. It scares me though. If you get known, there's some mean people out there who may take advantage, especially if you're disabled. First thing you know, your house gets broken into for money for heroin, and that kind of thing. Maybe we could keep my address out of it?"

"We'll talk to whoever reports your story about your safety concerns. We don't want anything bad to happen to you, Mrs. Dorst," said Max as he patted her hand.

"Well, something's got to give," Hannah said. "It's not only for me. I mean, there's lots of people out there struggling. In a country this rich you'd think everyone would be able to get the care we need, right?"

"When we're able to have a reporter talk with you, we'll have Max and Casey bring you to the office. Okay?"

Chapter 23

Back at the office, Tom found a message from Barry Ringer. He took a deep breath and returned the call.

"Barry, Tom Barrett here." He stopped there, fearing what Barry would say.

"Hi, Tom." Barry paused for what Tom thought was a beat too long.

"Well, things are better here," he said, and Tom was confused as to what took him so long. "Katharine woke up this morning. She's still groggy and confused, but she recognized her parents and me. She nodded when she saw us. Not talking yet, still has her trach tube in place, but she's able to move her arms and legs."

"Good signs, as you know," Tom said, relief in every syllable. "Doctors telling you anything?"

"They're still close-mouthed about what to expect. She's down in MRI right now. Maybe we'll know more after that. I'll call you."

"Anything you want from me?"

"No, can't think of anything concrete," Barry said. "I told Hunter and Jeff I was calling you and they say 'hi.' They're real troupers. They're with Hunter Senior and Julie, at Katharine's house."

Tom didn't know what else to say but he stayed on the line to try to gauge how Barry was doing. After a minute of silence, he decided simply to ask.

"How're you doing?"

"I'm kinda a mess," he said, voice trembling. "Sleeping's tough, worried as hell. Not much I can do here but I can't leave the hospital while she's this way. I need to be here for her when she's fully awake."

"Go to your gym and work your ass off, sweat a lot, and that'll help. Nothing like physical exertion to flush out the bad humors."

"Good idea. I haven't done that since she's been here. Thanks, Tom, from all of us."

"Barry, call me back in a couple of days when you know a little more from the doctors, okay?"

"Will do, Tom. I hope it'll be good news."

Tom speculated to himself about how much function she might have lost. Experience told him of wide variability. *Some never get full cognitive function back to an original state, can never go back to work, lose executive function. Some have peculiar changes in personality: manic behaviors or deep depression. What would it be like for Katharine?*

Chapter 24

"Dr. Barrett, this is Max. I got in touch with my sister. She referred me to Ruth Belsun on the Searchlight Team. She's willing to come here and talk with us."

"Fantastic! When?"

"Up to you. When are you available?"

"I'll clear my calendar for her anytime."

Ten minutes later Max called back.

"She can come in about two hours. Whadda ya think of that?"

"Pretty incredible. Think you can pick Hannah up and bring her here? Rent an SUV because she'll have trouble getting into your VW. I'm gonna ask one of our board members, Eileen Givens, if there's any way she could join us. She's a journalist and knows how that world works. See you."

Tom called Eileen.

"In two hours? Are you insane? Do you think I sit here waiting for your call?" Eileen said in her typical snarky way.

Tom's face flushed with embarrassment. *What was I thinking?*

"Sorry," he said. "I'm so excited about this interview I've lost all sense of reality. I'll let you know how it goes."

"I didn't say I wouldn't come," Eileen laughed. "I'll be there. But don't think this is gonna be my modus operandi. You call, and I jump!"

"Nobody's ever done that for me," Tom chuckled. "Thanks for jumping this time. I owe you one."

"You owe me two or three, but I'll settle for one."

Two hours later, Ruth Belsun, young, painfully thin and hyperactive, danced into the conference room where Eileen and Tom sat.

"Hi, I'm Tom Barrett. Thanks for coming. And I think you know Eileen Givens, right?"

"Eileen! Didn't recognize you when I rolled in. Good to see you again." Turning to Tom, Ruth said, "Eileen's one of my heroes. When she worked at the *Tribune,* I read every one of her columns." Eileen threw her a kiss.

Tom provided a general overview of Hannah's situation.

"So, she's a victim of the adalimumab saga," Ruth said. "I'm really pissed at the inhumanity in that company."

"You've seen this show?" Tom said.

"Anyone in the media who doesn't know this story should find another line of work. It's disgraceful what that company has done. And continues to do."

"Has Max told you what we at PharmaTruth do?"

"Some, but after I interview the patient -- what's her name -- I'd like to talk with you in more depth."

"Gladly. The patient's name is Hannah Dorst. Sweet woman," Tom said.

***

Ruth's shoulders slumped as she watched Max and Casey help Hannah Dorst maneuver her walker into the conference room. Her courageous exertion added even more motivation for Ruth to broadcast Hannah's story, take it as far as it would fly. After introducing everyone, Tom turned to Hannah.

"Mrs. Dorst, Ruth would like to hear about your experience with your arthritis, how long you've had to cope with it, and the problems you've had with getting prescriptions, the cost, and all that. I'll sit and listen while the two of you have your conversation. Tell us at any time if you need a break for any reason. Okay?"

"I'm ready anytime you are," she said to Ruth. "Do you care if I record what you say? I want to be sure I get it right," Ruth said.

"I've come this far. What harm can recording have? Sure, go ahead."

An hour later, Ruth turned off the recording device.

"Hannah, thank you so much for talking to me. I truly believe telling your story will help bring change."

"Thank you, Ruth. I hope so, and God bless you for doing this work." Hannah reached over and placed her hand on Ruth's arm. "Can I ask you something?"

"Anything, Hannah."

"You've been a reporter for a while. What happens when someone like me goes up against the bigwigs? You've probably gotten people mad at you. Do you ever get afraid someone might harm you for what you do?"

"Look at me, Hannah. I'm not thin for nothing. Sure, I get anxious when I write things about powerful people and corporations. Especially about healthcare reform. It gets political, too. I've been called a communist, a socialist and have been faced with threats that thankfully have never materialized. Here I am." She paused and looked at Hannah. "Are you scared?"

"I wish I were braver. Yeah, I'm plenty scared. I'm defenseless and live alone. And my neighborhood is not the safest in town. I got double locks on the door, but friends tell me if they want to get in, door locks won't stop 'em."

"Hannah, I won't print or divulge your address at any time. I can even refer to you simply as a Massachusetts resident, if that helps you to feel more comfortable. However, if it comes to congressional hearings, then you would have to give your name while testifying, but I doubt your address would be made public. But I'm not sure about that."

"Call me if you have any specific worries or if there are threats," Tom said. "PharmaTruth's head of security, George Logan, used to be a police officer. He'd know what to do. Also, call the local police station, Hannah, and ask them what kind of security system you should install. One that sends an alarm directly to the station. PharmaTruth will pay to get it installed. A small way to thank you for what you've done."

Chapter 25

Tom pressed the doorbell on Athens Street in South Boston. Yolanda Jefferson, his community representative on the board, had come along for this meeting.

"I wonder if Gwen Allen will have misgivings about a Black face at her door," Yolanda said. "You know, this is Southie. In the sixties there was a lot of trouble comin' outta this neighborhood during the bussing crisis. Course I wasn't even born then, ya know," she said with a smile.

"I don't know Gwen Allen, but there's been a lot of change in Southie since those days. My guess is she'll be glad to see both of us."

The speaker on the doorbell panel came on.

"Who is it?"

"Tom Barrett and Yolanda Jefferson from PharmaTruth."

A loud buzzing filled the alcove. When they got to Gwen's second floor apartment, her door was ajar. Tom knocked.

"Come on in. I'll be right with you."

The building's drab exterior had deceived Tom and Yolanda into thinking this was low-income housing. Contrary to expectations, her apartment was modern and well appointed. Gwen carried a tray with coffee and tea to the living room and greeted Yolanda and Tom warmly.

"Thanks for meeting with us," Tom said. Tom handed a newly minted brochure of PharmaTruth to Gwen.

"Just to give you a tangible piece of information about our organization. I hope we can help each other.

"So, please tell us about your experience."

Gwen unloaded her tale of unwitting addiction while Tom took notes. Yolanda gazed at her in sympathy. When she was through, Tom looked up from writing.

"Now for the big question, Gwen. Are you willing to share this with the press? Possibly with committees of legislators?"

"Absolutely! I want to see these bastards -- pardon my language -- exposed and punished," she said, her face reddening. "Anything I can do to insure that happens, I'm in."

"Here's how you can help: we have a reporter, name's Ruth Belsun, who's helping us put this into a front-page series for the Searchlight Team. Television stations will also pick this up. The Massachusetts Attorney General has already sued AH Pharmaceuticals. Another firm was found guilty in Boston for their criminal activity," Tom said. "They're being charged with bribes and kickbacks to physicians who prescribed spray fentanyl, a drug intended for cancer patients, for patients who had no cancer."

"Until this happened to me, I had no idea this was going on," Gwen said. "I consider myself well informed. But you know, when a headline doesn't involve you personally, you probably don't read the article.

"You can count on me," Gwen said with conviction. "I'm in this for the long haul."

"Thank you. Ruth Belsun will call you. We greatly appreciate your courage to come forward."

Chapter 26

Dina called George on her covert phone. "George, I need to catch you up. When would be a good time for us to meet?"

"You name it, I'll be there. Same place?"

Early next morning, Dina sat down across from George in Coffee Obsession. She looked around to be sure no one was watching them. Reassured, she turned to George.

In a low voice, passing a manila envelope to George, Dina said, "I'm giving you a copy of my notes so far. Just in case someone gets suspicious, and these get into the wrong hands. The notes describe Warner, in his own words, arranging for bribery of insurance execs with stocks of Cidal, in exchange for covering the drug, paying doctors to recommend the drug, and hoisting prices."

"These will go in a safe place," George said. "How're you feeling about this?"

"I feel dirty, but I signed on for it."

"Are you scared of Warner?"

"Not so far. But if he suspected I wasn't loyal to him I know he'd turn on me like a viper. He's a real predator, and I don't mean only a sexual predator. I'm convinced he'd attack anyone who threatened his pursuit of wealth."

"Does he know where you live?"

"I'm sure it's in my employment file in Human Resource Why?"

"Think about it. If he caught a whiff about what you're doing, you'd be in dangerous waters. Anywhere you could send your daughter to live?"

A chill of fear spread through Dina's body. It was like George had overheard her conversation with Warner when he asked about her daughter. She was jolted into awareness about possibly making Debbie a target. *Why haven't I thought of this sooner? How naïve.*

"What the hell is missing in my brain?" she said with a groan. "When I decided to take this on, I didn't think it through. I was so angry that this great new drug was a mere moneymaker for that selfish schmuck. If Cidal had been around when Mom was fighting postoperative infection, she might be alive."

"Your 'save the world' impulses might have clouded your thinking, so don't beat yourself up. You're in good company with that idealism. Now, though, you need to be more careful, look out for yourself and your daughter. Maybe you should get a new address."

"Move? How would that work? Move in the dark of night? And what about Debbie? We live two blocks from her school. She might have a problem getting there if we lived elsewhere." She took a deep breath. "You suppose she's at risk? If Warner wanted to get at me, he could have her kidnapped!"

"Let's not go there. That's unlikely. You're the one in danger if Warner gets rough. We need to protect *you*."

"You mean police? What would justify that? And wouldn't that arouse suspicion if they're already watching me?"

"I doubt they're watching you if you're reading Warner correctly. But a private detective keeping tabs on you would be a great prophylactic measure. I'll talk to Tom."

"How will I know?"

"I'll tell you. And Dina – what you're doing is important, and you're one courageous woman. I'll have your back."

"Thanks George, for being my guardian angel. I just wish I didn't need one."

"We all need one."

***

Dina stepped into the lobby of Pylea Pharmaceuticals with a new consciousness and new fear. She felt like an African steenbok, food for a range of predators lying in wait. She hadn't felt this until now and hoped it didn't show. On her desk was a note.

"See me as soon as you get in. Reggie."

At least he signed it "Reggie." Her heartbeat sped up, and her armpits were wet. What could he want? Her heels clicked on the hardwood floors as she approached his office. His door was closed. She knocked.

"Wait a minute; I'm on the phone," Warner barked.

Dina glanced at her reflection in the glass door. Her heart was still pounding, and her head felt light, but she didn't appear different. The door opened and he stood there, blank-faced, staring at her.

"Come on in," he said, not unfriendly, but not as patronizing as that morning after their liaison.

"How are you?" she said, wondering if she could discern sources of his grumpiness.

"Not good. This fucking liberal state is giving me fits. Newspapers and TV make my blood pressure go up, every morning. The AG's gone after Purdue and Insys, blaming them for this opioid epidemic. Not fair. People who get addicted, it's their own fault. It's like blaming tobacco companies for lung cancer or whisky makers for alcoholism."

Dina stifled a reply. *He's a classic denier. How much more proof does anyone need to believe that cigarettes cause lung cancer? That whisky can cause addiction to alcohol.* She tried not to listen as Warner continued to spew his hate in every direction. At least she wasn't an object of his scorn. She hoped she wouldn't be near him when he decided she was disloyal, a sworn enemy. She wondered about her notes being read.

"How is the promotional material coming along?"

"It's ready for your approval. Shall I print it out or should I send it by email?"

"Nothing by email anymore! Bring over a printed copy. And do it right now. I want to get going with this before the shit hits the fan altogether.

"Been talking to a couple of big hospitals in town and they're eager to get Cidal. When I mention the $500,000 cost, they don't sweat it. I told these two biggies I'd cut a deal with them if they praise the results publicly. They agreed. Their balls are on the block. The insurance companies have no choice but to pay up. They'll raise premiums to cover their costs anyhow, so it's no big deal to them."

Dina wondered how much more damning information she could learn if she became intimate with him. But prostitute herself? It was a sick thought that just because she was female, that's how to accomplish her goal. And then wouldn't that make him feel even more betrayed?

"You free tonight?"

What excuse could she invent? She can't talk about Debbie needing her. The last thing she wanted was to let Warner know anything about her.

"What do you have in mind?" she said, mildly flirtatious.

"Another night like Wednesday. We left a few dreams unfulfilled," he said suggestively.

Dina felt disgusted. *How very sweet to know that.*

"Same time? Same place?" she asked.

"Sounds delicious. See you then."

Dina was relieved that he seemed not to suspect anything, even as she was repulsed by having to spend more time with him; it would take much more effort to put him off. She went back to her office and called George on her private phone.

"George, had a chance to look at my notes?"

"Yeah, good stuff," he said. "Why are you calling? You okay?"

"I'm okay, but wondering how much more do we need? Is there a lawyer who could tell me how much is enough?"

"I'll run it by Tom and let you know."

"Looks like I have another date with Warner tonight. So, I'd like to know what's next."

After the call, Dina took the printed marketing plan to Warner's secretary, hoping not to encounter him. She handed the folder to Shelby.

Warner's door opened. "Bring it on in here," he said. "I'll read it right away."

She walked in, gave him the folder, and turned to leave.

"Sit down. I'll make my corrections, and you can take it back and edit it. Then return it and we'll send it right off to Burrer."

She sat down and picked up a travel magazine. In the back pages were ads for villas in the Caribbean. One ad caught her eye because it had some scribbling on it. It was an isolated gated community in Trinidad. So, this was where he wanted to live out his dream of white sands, freedom from care, and awful to contemplate, her presence.

"Okay, this is great. I've added a couple of things. Make these additions and bring it back, give it to Shelby. See you later, around 5:30. You know where."

***

They met at his car and went to dinner. During the early part of the evening, he unveiled another look into his corrupt world.

"I have some stock guys who're gettin' a bunch of investors to buy Cidal stock at its current value. Before it spikes, after it's released for sale."

"I don't know much about stocks," Dina said, "but isn't that what they call 'insider trading?'"

"Yeah, that's what the outsiders call it. We insiders call it "business as usual."

Her entree was truly delicious, so it took some acting for Dina to stop eating and begin to push the food around on her plate. It took about ten minutes, since he was sermonizing about the stock market, before he tuned in to her strategy.

"Not pleased with the food? Waiter!" Warner shouted.

"Oh no. It's not that," Dina said. "My stomach has been feeling queasy all day. I thought maybe drinking that ginger ale would settle it, but I'm afraid it's gotten worse. I wanted to get together, so I pushed myself, but I'm afraid that I'll be in a worse situation soon." Dina did feel awful, this wasn't a total stretch of the truth. Warner was studying her.

She looked him directly in the eyes. "I'm sorry, but could you please drive me back to the office? Actually, I don't want to get sick in your beautiful car; I'll get an Uber."

"Good point. If you're that sick…but it's damn disappointing," Warner said, seeming more irritated than sympathetic.

Dina went home with another morsel of damning evidence. She was desperate for this ruse to end soon. At least the waiter had put her food in a doggy bag.

***

George, Tom, Dina and someone Dina hadn't met before gathered in Tom's office at seven AM on Saturday morning. Their agenda was simple: compile a list of Reginald Warner's and Pylea Pharmaceuticals' misdeeds that Dina had discovered in meetings with her boss. Dina also hoped they could determine whether she could quit her distasteful job.

Tom made the introductions. "Dina, this is David Longstreet, a board member and lawyer for plaintiffs in drug cases. David, Dina's been documenting information about Pylea Pharmaceuticals and their new drug, Cidal. It's a much-needed drug that will revolutionize treatment of resistant post-operative infections. Not on the market yet but soon to be released. Dina, we need to analyze what you've heard from Warner, what can be used in court. Can you tell us what you know?"

"I looked over my notes and came up with six points. Shall I begin??"

"Yes, thank you," Tom said. "David will tell us which points are legally useful."

"Okay, here goes. Number one is price inflation. The actual cost of manufacturing Cidal is very low, considering its importance. But Warner and his so-called Executive Council are pricing it at $500,000 per treatment kit."

"For each patient?" David asked.

"For each and every patient. That's why Warner thinks he'll be one of the richest guys in the world. Shall I go on?

"Can't wait to hear how you can top that one," Tom mumbled, already feeling his heart rate go up, his adrenalin surging.

"Number two is that Pylea's Executive Council members repeatedly say that profit is the only important thing."

"That's a non-starter," David said. "That's modus operandi for any business, especially, in my experience, the drug industry. They like to advertise what they do is for the good of the patient, but it's not. Go on."

"Number three, Warner told me he conspired with two of the biggest U.S. health insurance companies -- Old Forge and Winger -- to pay whatever the price, in exchange for Pylea stock. It's cheap now, before the drug's released, but anticipated to shoot up rapidly after it's introduced."

David briskly took notes as Dina spoke. "He can't do that," David said. "Those companies' books have to be audited, and that kind of deal would be exposed easily."

"He's aware of that. Stock would be purchased by the wives or other relatives so it wouldn't show on the company books," Dina said. "Oh, another thing. When he went to the men's room while we were at dinner, he left his cell phone on the table. I jotted down the number and the carrier. I've also gotten his private email address, the one he does these schemes on."

"You're a genius," Longstreet exclaimed. "Those can be subpoenaed and will probably have evidence we'll need to prove what you've been telling us."

Tom was clicking his pen repeatedly and abruptly rose from his chair. He ran his hand through his hair, walked to the window and paced around his desk. Dina looked at George, the only calm person in the room, as usual.

"Tom, think you ought to sit down and relax," George said. "This is only the beginning. It's gonna get worse. This is only the first of many cases."

Dina gazed around the room. "Should I continue?"

"Press on," David said.

"Number four, this is a good one: Bribing two famous infectious disease specialists from prominent Boston hospitals to promote the drug vigorously at national and international conferences where they're featured speakers. Reward for this: full expenses paid, month-long family vacations in Hawaii."

"Jeez, can't they afford that on their own?" Tom said, disgusted.

"Number five: getting hundreds of sales representatives to push Cidal for EVERY post-op patient. They're calling this 'prophylaxis' and telling doctors and hospitals this will end infectious disease threats in their hospitals. And as a pharmacologist, I can tell you this means that, faster than would be natural, this med will lose its efficacy and stronger resistant strains of bacteria will emerge. So, they're intentionally corrupting the benefits of Cidal, for profit.

"And number six: insider trading of Cidal stock."

Sunlight streamed into the room as Dina finished. No one broke the silence for several minutes. David continued writing on his yellow legal pad. Tom resumed clicking his pen. George closed his eyes to the sun and felt warmed as it moved onto his face. Finally, David looked up with a smile.

"This is dynamite. Dina, what a job you've done."

"Am I finished? Can I quit?"

"I hate to say this, but quitting suddenly could negate what you've already accomplished," George said. "If you quit abruptly, Warner may figure you've been up to something and quickly take steps to cover up his actions. We need an exit strategy that won't trigger suspicion, or revenge. I'm afraid we need you to hang in there a while longer."

"How much longer? You don't realize how much I hate that man! And I don't know how long I'll be able to put off his advances."

"We really can't put her in this situation," Tom said.

"Absolutely, I'll get on it right away. Hang tight, and we'll devise a way out for you. It might be dramatic. I don't know…I'll give it some serious thought," George said, feeling guilty, like a chess master who'd failed to plan the winning strategy.

"We need to rescue Dina from this assignment as soon as possible," Tom said. "Could she claim a fatal illness? Go missing?"

Tom strained to find a way to extricate Dina from this dilemma.

"Let me think, just for a day or two," George said. "I'll come up with a plan."

Chapter 27

Dolores handed Tom a message when he walked into his office, an unusual gesture that suggested urgency.

It was from Barry Ringer. Tom closed the door to this office and called.

"Hi Tom, you told me to call when we had more medical results. The good news is that her MRI is nearly normal. The not so good news is that she seems a bit different than the pre-accident Katharine."

"What do you mean, Barry? In what way is she different?"

"Well, she recognizes everyone, but she seems euphoric, laughs a lot, but it seems to me out of place. Maybe it's she's so relieved to be alive and without any paralyses or speech problems. I don't know. It's jarring."

"It sounds like a change in what we call 'affect.'"

"Yes, yes that's the exact word the doctors are using. I don't understand what that is. Can you explain it?"

"Affect is like mood. Some people have what we call a 'flat' affect, that is, they don't respond with any change in expression. Some people have 'inappropriate' affect, which is what you seem to be describing. That may be transient as she recovers. Remember, she's had a significant head injury. She's lucky not to have more serious sequelae."

"She's going to be discharged in a few days to the rehab unit where she'll begin physical therapy and what they call occupational therapy. The unit is right here at the hospital."

"Did you take my advice and go to the gym?"

"I did and it helped a lot. But I'm feeling kinda down. She's not the same person I knew."

"You probably should get some therapy yourself. You've been through a lot too."

"Yes, I have an appointment for that. The doctors and nurses here suggested that as they watched me get more worried as the days progressed."

"Do you know when I could either talk to her or email her? Or should I just write her an old-fashioned letter?"

"She has a phone now," he said, and gave Tom the number. "She'd love to hear from you."

"Things okay with the boys?"

"They're doing better than I am. They come in regularly to see their mom, and they have a good time together."

"Great. Thanks, Barry, I'll give her a call. And take care of yourself."

Tom immediately called. Katharine answered after the first ring.

"Hi Katharine, it's Tom Barrett. How are you getting along?"

"Oh Tom, how wonderful of you to call. I'm doing marvelously. The doctors are pleased with me, and I'm pleased with them. I'm ready to go home any day now." She chattered on for a couple of minutes before Tom could get a word into the conversation.

"Barry told me you were going into rehab soon. Is that right?"

"Oh yes, but that won't take long. I'm ready to roll! I feel great."

Tom heard exactly what Barry had described. Her affect was inappropriately joyful. His hope was that this would be replaced by a more tranquil mood once she began physical and occupational therapy.

"Tom, I need to go for some kind of test now. They're waiting for me. I'll call you back tomorrow, okay? Thanks so much for calling."

"Bye, Katharine. Talk to you soon."

The call was not as reassuring as he'd hoped. He understood Barry's take on it and it was worrisome. He recalled one of his mentors saying that, after a head injury and coma, people "are never the same." *Loss of brain cells leaves its traces behind.* Memories of his own flashbacks, temper outbursts, impatience—and his assault on Cynthia—flooded back. Without warning, his hand swept up to his face as tears dripped from his eyes and a deep sob rose from his chest. *People are never the same.*

Chapter 28

Senator Rafferty's Chief of Staff Noah Brinkley briefed his boss about PharmaTruth before arranging another meeting with George.

"On their website they say their mission is to 'shine a light on questionable practices of pharmaceutical companies.' What they've done, according to their coordinator of volunteers, was to receive over 7,000 hits on their website. People complaining about the price of their prescriptions, confusion about generics, insurance coverage, and their inability to talk to their doctors about any of this."

Rafferty nodded in understanding as Noah told him what he'd learned by talking with PharmaTruth Board members who represented practically every aspect of medical care.

"Impressive board talent and diversity," the senator said. "Move forward with exploring this."

"Yes, sir," Noah said and left to set up a second meeting.

"Hello Mr. Logan. The senator wants to meet Dr. Barrett. Please ask him to come speak with him," Noah told George, the tone suggesting this was not a request, but an expectation.

"Yes, of course; Tom and I have already discussed this. He looks forward to meeting Senator Rafferty." George knew how to be deferent when it served his purposes. "Two questions: When? And is there an agenda?"

"How about next Wednesday at two PM? And no agenda, this is simply a get acquainted meeting."

***

The following Wednesday, after lunch at Faneuil Hall, Tom and George walked to the JFK Federal Building, went through security and found an elevator. They were shown into Senator Rafferty's conference room.

"The senator is on a phone call, but he'll be along shortly," Noah said, shaking hands with them. "Dr. Barrett, I'm Noah Brinkley, Senator Rafferty's chief of staff. Thanks for coming. We're excited about the work you're doing and hope we can help."

"Thanks. We're pleased to be here and share that hope," Tom said and smiled.

As he spoke, Rafferty walked briskly into the room. "Greetings!"

Noah made the introductions, and the senator took over the meet and greet.

"Dr. Barrett, Mr. Logan, thanks for coming. I was just talking with Congresswoman Eva Brill of Ohio about your work. She and I may introduce companion bills to address some of your concerns about drug companies. It's a tricky business as you know, but I think we can cobble together some language for a bill that will address some of the problems."

"I'd be interested in consulting on that effort," Tom said. "We also have board members who are experts in their fields, and they'd be eager and willing to help."

"We'll need every bit of help we can get. I've been appalled by the tactics of Purdue and Insys," Rafferty said. "Legislation can do a number of things, but lawsuits like those against Purdue and Insys should be powerful disincentives to such practices."

"What bothers me most about Insys Therapeutics," Tom said, taking up a subject that made his blood pressure readings soar, "is the news that came out of the racketeering trial in Boston. That Insys trained employees to lie to insurers about previous failed pain meds so that insurers would approve the use of Subsys. And lying about patients having acute, ongoing cancer when, in fact, some cancers were in remission, or even cured, for as long as twenty years." Tom saw George looking at him with raised eyebrows. He took a couple of deep breaths, barely able to heed Kumar's advice to remain calm and not go off half-cocked. *People are never the same.*

Rafferty's frown deepened as he listened to Tom.

"I know how you feel, Dr. Barrett. I've been around the block in my career, both in the Senate and before that when I ran our state's Housing and Community Development Department. I've seen a lot of bad behavior by business and by government employees alike." He folded his hands on the table and turned his steady blue eyes on Tom. "But the current crop of crooks is by far the worst. And I think it's a direct result of our national leadership's sorry role models."

George thought about Dina's work in Pylea. Another example of a corrupt company whose tactics were unconscionable in so many ways. Should he bring that up? No, the case against Pylea was for the Massachusetts Attorney General to pursue.

"Senator, please come to one of our board meetings so board members can detail the issues we're addressing," Tom said.

"Absolutely. I'll need a mountain of evidence as Brill and I craft our bills. May I bring Noah and an administrative assistant? Three sets of ears capture more than my failing hearing," he laughed.

As George and Tom left the Federal Building, they dared not look at one another for fear of bursting out in exhilarated laughter. The meeting with Rafferty couldn't have gone better. Once they were back at their office, they closed Tom's door and embraced, laughing and giving each other high fives.

When they came back to reality, George said, "Need to talk to you about Dina."

"What's wrong?"

"Nothing's wrong. I want to keep it that way. She's gotten a lot of incriminating stuff on that creep Warner and others in that rat's nest," George said. "But I'm worried he's gonna figure out what she's up to and take some unsavory steps. I'm also concerned about her seventeen-year-old daughter. So is Dina."

"Any reason to think she's under suspicion?"

"Not yet. But one false step and that could change. I want to take preemptive action to insulate her from harm."

"Such as?"

"I think, at the very least, put a detective on her to watch for sketchy conduct around her house and to keep an eye on her. She's been going on dinner dates with Warner in the line of duty and she wants to end it before she's put in a situation she can't get out of. There'll be radioactive fallout when she tells him her interest in him is over. Or when she walks out of her job."

"Do we have enough dirt on him?"

"I think so. What a jury thinks of evidence like this is anybody's guess, but she's got a lot."

"Do we have enough so we can afford to have her stop?" Tom asked.

George glued his eyes on Tom. "The issue is: can *she* afford to continue? She's the one risking her neck. I don't think it's a question of whether *we* can afford it. I'm a little surprised you put it that way," George said.

"You're right, I'm sorry," Tom said, shoulders sagging. His previous exhilaration drained from his face. "Of course, that was my first thought after our meeting: get her out of there. I don't know why I backpedaled."

"Okay, now, don't get all guilty on me. I'm the one to blame for getting too personally involved with her safety."

"Yeah, well sometimes I get so worked up going after these jerks, I forget about sacrifices other people are making."

Tom paused a moment, his thoughts left the room and settled on a memory of Cynthia, terrorized by one of his violent outbursts before his medication had worked its magic.

"You decide how best to protect Dina. You know what she's doing for us better than I."

George quickly went to his office, closed the door, and hurriedly called Dina. He paced his office while her phone rang and rang with no response.

"Dammit, answer! Where are you?" he said as he fidgeted with his keyboard.

Finally, her answering message came on. He left a curt message hoping it didn't sound angry or nervous. He worried he'd dropped the ball and waited too long to ensure Dina's well-being.

Dusk blotted out his view of the State House and his watch confirmed what his stomach told him – dinner was needed. The physical exertion of walking to Legal Seafood calmed him and once he'd eaten his spicy deep-fried fish and chips, his digestive temper tantrum ended. As he finished wiping the oil from his fingers, his phone buzzed. It was Dina.

"Dina!" he shouted. "You okay?"

"Well, yeah, *I'm* okay. But you sounded agitated. What's wrong?"

"Just frustrated I couldn't reach you. Not to worry. What's happening?"

"Another date is set with you-know-who for this evening."

"Can we meet tomorrow, same time, same place? I want to discuss an exit strategy for you."

"Oh yay! Can't wait to be done with this. I'm gonna need extra therapy when this is over with."

"See you tomorrow then. Sorry about tonight's assignment."

He knew he'd do nothing but worry about her until he saw her walk into Coffee Obsession twelve hours from now.

***

"You're late!" Warner yelled when she swung her legs into the car. "Where the hell have you been?"

Dina looked at her watch. "I'm five minutes late, for goodness' sake. Why are you so upset?"

"I don't like to wait for anyone, even you," he fumed as he backed up and lit a cigarette filling the car with pungent smoke. "I'm hungry and thirsty – for food and for something else that's satisfying, with a twist."

Dina's stomach did a flip-flop. *What does that mean?*

They ate in silence for a while. Dina's heartbeat pulsed steadily in her ears. She didn't like his mood or attitude. Does he suspect something? Or is he just feeling threatened by the Purdue and Insys revelations? What else could be bugging him?

Tension prompted her to engage Warner in conversation.

"How do you think the conversations with the hospitals and insurance people are going?"

"I don't want to talk about business," he said in a low voice. He kept glancing at her in a new way. "I've known a lot of women who come off as gentle and innocent who turn out to be the wildest in the bedroom. Are you one of those?"

Dina, taken aback by this shift in his mood, decided to deflect his question and took a new tack.

"I noticed a magazine in your office with a resort in Trinidad circled. You planning on a trip there?"

"I'd like to take you with me, not only for a vacation, but for a longer time. Interested?"

"Never been to Trinidad. Sounds like a fabulous place."

"Going together would make it fabulous. I've been there several times. You'd love the place I have in mind." His face softened as he gazed at her.

"Well, I'll sure think about it." She hoped this would be sufficient encouraging, not too off-putting. They finished dinner and, without even asking, he drove into the parking garage under his condo.

"Come on up," he said. "We can have a nightcap. No more excuses. I'm getting the idea that you're one of those hysterical females who tease and tease but never deliver."

"Don't think that. And it's not very romantic of you to say something like that. Of course, I'll come upstairs with you."

The door to Warner's condo testified to its previous life as an apartment, with the hall dotted with separate condo entries. The hallway took an oblique turn at one end, giving the impression that the building had been constructed to fit an odd space. As Dina followed Warner through the door of his living space, she had no question that this was his apartment, as the stale odor of cigarettes clung to every surface. The unit was populated by furniture easily recognized as rented. The art on the walls shouted that it came from a hotel going-out-of-business sale. Nothing in the condo suggested anything personal about the owner.

Warner pretended to show her around the condo. When they came to his bedroom, Dina's stomach tightened, but she worried that he would discover her game. She stood in the doorway.

"So, this is where you rest from your business power plays?" Dina said. She hoped they'd have a drink and maybe he'd fall asleep if she stalled long enough.

"I'm going to show you one of my favorite power plays," he said, moving to his closet. "Come inside the room. What are you standing there for?"

"Where's the nightcap you promised? A man with your fine taste must have some amazing cognac."

"We're done with imbibing. Time for play," Warner said moving towards the bed, and to Dina's dismay, he was holding leather straps.

"No, no! I don't do those things!" she said with as much force as she could, stepping backwards. A quick sideways glance located her purse on the sideboard a couple of feet away.

"You'll do what I want," he growled. "I've waited long enough, wined and dined you. Who do you think you're playing with? Get down on the bed."

"That's not how a gentleman talks," Dina said and rushed to grab her purse. Frantically, she groped inside to find her Mace canister. *Where is it? It was here this morning!*

"I think this date is over," she said as she dashed to her coat, still rummaging in her purse for her Mace canister. He jumped up and chased her just as she grasped the canister.

"Where do you think you're goin'?" he yelled, jumping up and chasing her.

Just as he was about to put hands on her, Dina's fingers closed on the canister. She whipped it out and aimed it at him, pressing the valve.

The spray glanced off his face but enough hit the mark so that he staggered, screaming obscenities as he backed into the bathroom and doused his face with water. Dina dashed out of the apartment, slamming the door shut. She didn't know if she hoped the corridor was empty or occupied.

Adrenalin spiking, Dina looked wildly both ways. *Which way did we come from?*

"Bitch!" she heard Warner screaming.

Dashing to the right, she turned and saw him staggering out of the condo, looking left and right. He spotted her.

Oh my God! Which way to the parking garage? Is there another exit?

Ripping her phone out of her purse she called 911, stuttering into the receiver. She ran down the hall. With amazing alacrity for man his age, Warner pursued her. Seeing the door to the stairwell, she careened into it, skipping stairs going down, praying not to fall. Warner didn't follow her. That must mean he took the elevator and would be waiting for her on the first floor. She was at level two and left the stairwell into an identical corridor as the one above. *Which way from here? Where are the police cars?* Not a single flashing light of an approaching cruiser was in sight.

Dina ran and found another stairwell. *Where to go? Should I go up, fool Warner if he's waiting for me on the first floor? That's only going to buy me a tiny bit of time until the police get here. Maybe he's realized that I stopped going down the stairs and he's heading up the stair to me right now. Where the hell are the cops? What else can I do? George. Call George. He'll know what to do. Come rescue me, George!*

"Urgently she whispered to Siri, "Call George."

"Calling George," Siri responded. *Oh my God, I hope he can't hear Siri.*

"George? I'm at Warner's condo and he's chasing me around the hallways. I need help!"

"Quick, the address. You caught me in my car, so I can come immediately."

"Ninety-six Eliot Street, Cambridge, off Mass Ave."

"Stay on the line," George instructed her. "It happens that I'm not far from there. I'll call 911 again on my other phone, but keep moving, don't try to hide." The line went silent, then Dina heard George's voice, "You there?"

"Yeah, I'm here. I feel frozen, don't know whether to go up or down. I'm not sure which stairwell he'll come out of. I don't see Warner right now. But hurry!"

"I am. Warner may not want to be found out. Maybe he'll retreat to his unit. Was he very drunk?"

"Not so much. In a foul mood, though. I wonder if he's on to me. Oh my God! There he is at the end of this corridor -- he sees me! I'm heading downstairs. He's about 100 feet away."

"There should be an exit door at the bottom of the stairs. Move fast; since you have a jump on him, you'll be able to make it. I'm almost there. Get to the first floor and come out. I'll find you."

Sirens, finally! Two police cars arrived with lights flashing. George pulled in right behind them. Dina popped out of the ground level stairwell and ran towards George. Warner was nowhere to be seen. George pulled Dina aside.

"Don't tell the cops who's been chasing you. We can't let them know what this is about. Tell them you were at a bar and this guy, you don't know his name, and you started talking and one thing led to another. He invited you to his condo and tried to assault you. Tell them you were naïve, thought he was an alright guy, you should have known better. When they ask you for an apartment number or floor tell them you don't remember. When they ask you for more information and whether you want to have them investigate further, just play dumb, thank them for coming and say you just want to go home with me."

After everything transpired as George had said it would, Dina went with him to his car. The cops dispersed and Warner apparently went back to his condo, dodging any interactions with police.

George took Dina home. Debbie heard the front door open but was busy studying her iPad and at first didn't look up. When she did, the sight of her mom, looking disheveled and upset, coming in with a Black man she didn't know, overwhelmed her with fear and confusion.

Dina saw her worry and quickly said, "This is my friend, George."

"Nice to meet you," George said, warmly smiling at her. He was so sick of having to reduce anxiety in the white people he met. But looking at Dina, he could understand her concern. She did look a wreck.

"I need a Scotch to settle my nerves," Dina said. "Want one, George?" He nodded yes and she poured them drinks and slumped into the couch. Debbie just stood there, completely flummoxed.

"Debbie, let me fill you in on what your mother's been up to," Dina said with a sigh. "You know my new job at Pylea? Well, I've been working there to get facts on their illegal activities to give to a group that George works for, called PharmaTruth."

Debbie was so bewildered she couldn't find words to respond. She was incredulous as her mother told her about what she'd been doing. Her prissy straight arrow mother, doing things she could never have imagined. With widened eyes she looked back and forth between her mother and George, who nodded sympathetically. When Dina finished explaining, George spoke up.

"That brings us to a decision point, Dina. It's obvious you can't go back to work at Pylea. And since they know where you live, you're gonna have to move, right away." He looked at Debbie as he said this since he knew this was a big load of change for her. "Both of you need to pack some clothes, your devices, anything you can't live without, and we'll check you into a temporary place to live safely until we can find something more permanent. Dina, do you own this place or rent?"

"Own it with the bank. Do I have to sell it?"

"Sell our house, Mom?" Debbie said, alarmed.

"We can discuss that later. Right now, we need to get you two out of harm's way. Warner's gotta be hopping mad and will retaliate, for sure. We can take no chances. Tonight was a close call. We can't afford any more."

An hour later they were stuffed into George's car with all their portable necessary belongings, headed for a motel. Debbie wept and Dina tried comforting her. George realized he had not become Debbie's favorite person for making them move precipitously, but at least they were safe.

"I doubt you'll need to call me again tonight, but I'm available if you do. I hope you get some sleep," George said. "Debbie, I'm sorry about this, but it'll work out. This place is only for tonight, and tomorrow we'll help find you and your mom a house to rent close to your school."

"George, thanks for rescuing me," Dina said. "I never thought anything like this would ever happen to me. I've had a boring life until tonight."

"Never know what's gonna happen, do we?"

***

Back at his condo, Warner seethed with anger. "I'll get even with that bitch," he said, looking into his mirror to check on his reddened eyes. "She'll pay for this!"

Chapter 29

Sitting in the PharmaTruth conference room in the morning, waiting to watch the next act of, "The Senator and The Board," George felt relieved he'd been able to snatch Dina from an uncertain fate last night. He worried what Warner might try to do in retaliation. Looking around at the board members and their guests, it was a worry compounded by uneasiness about prematurely cultivating a relationship with Rafferty and rushing Tom into one, too. *Was I presumptuous to do that? No politician is totally clean. Isn't that a given? Just need to stay tuned into my gut instincts.*

"Before I turn the meeting over to Reed Burseik, let me welcome Senator Rafferty and Representative Brill," Tom said. "By the way, we need to thank George Logan for making the original contact with Senator Rafferty. This meeting springs out of his initiative." Tom's words reassured George that maybe he'd not been so presumptuous after all.

"Senator Rafferty and Representative Brill are contemplating writing legislation – companion bills for the Senate and Congress -- addressing issues we've often discussed. Senator, Congresswoman, we're pleased you're here. We hope to forge a continuing alliance that will bring about needed change.

"Reed, will you lead this discussion?"

"Thanks Tom. Let me introduce the board members." He handed a list to Brill and Rafferty and asked each board member to say a few words. He noted that Rafferty's aide busily wrote on a yellow legal pad.

"Now that we're acquainted, let's take these issues one at a time," Burseik said. "The first item is pricing. Some drugs are wildly expensive, some are not fully covered by insurance, some not covered at all."

Peter Smalley raised his hand.

"As a former CEO of a pharmacy chain, I witnessed the mysterious ways pharmaceutical companies set drug prices. Insurance is the phantom payer for many drugs, so most consumers, and even pharmacists have no idea what the true price is. One thing's for sure -- consumers are the last consideration. When uninsured people see what they must fork over for medicines they need, they often leave them on the pharmacy counters. It's hard to give an accurate number to those walkaways, but I know it happens frequently."

"Something else is happening," said Hans Oberschmidt, "and if you're not already aware of it, I'll let you in on an open secret: several companies have been sued for violating anti-trust laws and delaying lower cost generics from finding their way into the marketplace. Some settlements are sizable. One was a half-billion dollars in fines. But -- and this is my point -- costs of these fines are built into pricing or covered by insurance policies carried by the drug companies. They know the number of suits resulting in large fines is small, so they gamble they won't get caught."

"As a practicing internist, what bothers me is price gouging for drugs needed for survival," Dr. Berman said. "Remember when pricing for EpiPen, that life-saving drug for anaphylaxis, was suddenly jacked up astronomically? Has anyone here ever been stung by a hornet? If you're allergic to hornet stings and you have no EpiPen, you're a goner. Raising the price of EpiPen made big headlines, but makers of other drugs sneakily raise prices gradually, avoiding that kind of news splash. Raising drug prices like that has a similar effect on people who depend on drugs for their very existence. It increases their vulnerability considerably."

"So, the first area of proposed legislation should relate to drug prices," Burseik said. "Let's move on to advertising and marketing."

"As a journalist, I'm alarmed at how the media promotes drugs. TV ads are confusing," Eileen Givens said. They don't even tell you what diseases the advertised drugs are intended for. They never mention cost, partly because the ads are produced by national advertising agencies and prices vary in different locales. But more importantly, they don't want the consumer to know anything about the money that third-party insurers are paying. The only thing you see are dozens of deliriously happy people in ordinary daily activities. And disclaimers go on for almost as long as the ads do."

"What annoys me most," Yolanda Jefferson said, "is how ads always end with 'ask your doctor.' When I ask my doctor about a drug I've seen on TV, she scorns the ads. Says they're misleading, simplistic, and imply that patients are carbon copies of one another and that one size fits everyone."

"Who is *she*?" one of the aides whispered to the other.

"The list says she is a community representative," the other aide murmured.

"Until recently," Yolanda said, "women weren't included in many studies. Drug companies claim they can't risk including possible pregnant women in studies, and children are omitted from studies using the excuse that there could be risks to the growing, developing child.

"Black people are also routinely excluded, the claim being they're not cooperative. No wonder! After the Tuskegee syphilis studies, the Henrietta Lacks story, and countless other abuses of Black people in medical studies, why should they trust anyone asking them to be in a clinical trial? Consequently, drug trials exclude groups of people in a capricious way."

"Most countries don't allow direct-to-consumer advertising," David Longstreet said. "Telling patients they need to decide what drug they should take is disgraceful. Lay people can't make decisions like this, that's why they go to doctors. Even doctors are ignorant of a lot of drugs advertised on TV. Occasionally patients will insist they get a drug they've seen advertised and some doctors will cave and prescribe that drug. It takes too long to discuss the complexities of drug actions. Pressure's on for doctors to show large numbers of visits. Time-consuming education of patients about the nuances of drug actions and interactions, something the best doctors used to do, impedes efficiency."

"What else can be said about advertising?" Burseik asked.

"A problem I see, as a pharmacologist," said Dr. Arnhold, "is that pharmaceutical companies regularly change a tiny radical on a drug and then market it as 'new and improved,' when, in fact, it's the same old drug whose patent has run out. It's what we call 'old wine in new bottles,' or the more recent term 'evergreening.' But for the drug companies, a new patent is born that will last several more years insuring a monopoly and ever-rising price tag on their drug."

"I'm outraged by the enormous cost of advertising and marketing," Hans Oberschmidt, the canny economist, was now speaking. "Pick up any medical journal and there are dozens of pages of advertising, in gaudy color with smiling attractive models, all under 30, of course, or handsome smiling older people engaged in oh-so-happy activities. Following this are full pages of small print -- side effects and precautions -- that no one reads. Popular magazines do the same thing. Advertising piles on huge costs."

"We'll put advertising and marketing as our second focus, but this is gonna be tricky. Lots of questions here about restraint of trade and free speech." Burseik said as he wrote on the whiteboard. "These categories need to be developed, but what's next on our list?"

Dr. Berman raised his hand. "Drug companies manipulate prescribing behavior by practicing doctors, like me. Drug reps come to my office to 'educate' me about their company's drugs, plying me with samples and inaccurate and incomplete information about their wares," he said with disgust. "Most docs welcome samples since they can give them to needy patients. But doctors are human, and they prescribe these drugs because they're familiar and a drug rep has been 'good enough' to supply samples."

Bill Gould, the psychiatrist from Belmont, jumped in. "Drug houses also push 'educational events,' trips on cruise ships and vacations in luxurious resorts. They deploy elaborate displays of promotional materials in exhibit halls at medical conferences and hire prominent doctors known as 'key opinion leaders' as paid speakers at these events, to mold perceptions of particular drugs," Gould said. "These KOLs advocate using their sponsoring company's products. They're paid to do this. How much varies, but you can bet it's worth their while to be prostitutes for drug houses. These KOLs may be true believers in drugs they're pushing, but they have long ago lost any trace of objectivity."

"Is there evidence this makes a difference in prescribing habits of doctors?" Francis Boyle, the lawyer from Chicago whose background was in defending pharmaceutical companies, interjected.

"Absolutely," Berman said. "It's been studied. There's a direct link between these activities and particular drug sales. Drug houses themselves study this and have concluded it's worth continuing."

"And what would it take to get our hands on *those* studies? George said, knowing that no answer would come.

After a pause and a wry smile as an answer to George's rhetorical questions, Burseik said, "So, number three on our list is 'manipulation of prescribing behavior, eh? I think one or two more should round out our list of mountains to climb."

"How about manipulation of research?" Rick Levensohn, a scientist studying opioid addiction asked. "Some drug companies conduct in-house research and only publish findings favorable to their products. They bury negative results. Then there's another problem: companies designing studies, deciding on variables, patient populations studied, so-called inclusion/exclusion criteria, and so on."

Rafferty and Brill were gripped by this discussion. Their aides took notes furiously. Senator Rafferty was the first to speak after board members paused.

"May we count on you folks to appear before our committees to answer questions from committee members? I'll warn you, some questions will be hostile, very confrontational."

The group nodded in agreement. "Moreover, we're ready to give you or your representatives as much information about these matters as you need," Dr. Arnhold said. "This includes research articles with scientifically derived data, not the stuff that's thrown around at partisan rallies by politicians bought by drug houses. Voters need facts to decide which candidate will come through for them."

"I may be one of only a handful of conservative representatives who can say I've never taken a penny from the pharmaceutical industry," Congresswoman Brill said, with a little edge in her voice. "This issue is one close to my heart and to my constituency. I hear daily from people in my district about drug costs, access to needed drugs, all the things we've heard about today, in this room. I'm ready and eager to get some legislation through to alleviate...no, eliminate...the unfairness in this industry. So, I'm ready to press on with this".

"As I'm sure you know," Senator Rafferty added, "national elections are coming. Being on the side of the people against big Pharma is not only morally right but it'll help with the election. But the other side is getting an avalanche of donations from pharma and health insurance companies. We're pretty sure our side will come out well, but one never knows. Voters can be swayed at the last minute by propaganda, prevarications or just plain lies. With interference from foreign powers a lot of misinformation can go viral. So be sure to vote, get involved with the pols supporting this agenda, and keep your fingers crossed."

Tom looked at his watch. Time to end it.

"Thanks to Senator Rafferty and Congresswoman Brill for coming," he said. "We're here to help in any way we can as you take this on. You know it won't be easy or quick, nothing worth doing is. When I'm impatient for quick solutions I remind myself of women's suffrage, civil rights, LGBTQ progress. It takes chipping away until some balance is reached between profits the drug industry deserves and what's best for patients.

"Board members, we're not done. Take a break, but please stay for the rest of our meeting item in thirty minutes. We have Ruth Belsun, lead reporter for the Searchlight Team at the *Boston Register*, coming."

After they filed out, Tom clapped George on the shoulder.

"Thanks. This was your doing.

"On a different note, did you get Dina situated in a safe place?"

George thought about Dina and Debbie. Where should they go that would be safe? Should he find a realtor for her? Is that part of his job? He worried that his concern about Dina was getting beyond his role as a security guy, but he saw her as so vulnerable.

"Yes, for now," George said. "I just talked with her. We're looking for something with more space, a real house. Her daughter hates me for making them move, but they're safer where they are. I'm worried about what Warner will do."

"Are we providing surveillance?"

"Oh, yeah. 24/7. Must be done."

"We need to get her notes into a form where they can be presented in proceedings. We need to get her in touch with a lawyer."

***

Having long board meetings was not to everyone's liking but getting everyone to return was impractical and expensive. Having another meeting was mitigated by having two key legislators attend, symbolic of PharmaTruth's potential political clout.

"Quite a banner day for us," Burseik said when they reconvened. "First, a senator and a congresswoman, now Ruth Belsun. Eileen, would you like to introduce Ruth to the group?"

"Ruth Belsun needs no introduction to most of you," Eileen Givens said. "She's a Pulitzer Prize-winning journalist who's done some of the best investigative reports in Boston and Massachusetts over the last decade. Having been a reporter myself, let's not prolong the introduction and cut to the chase. Ruth, tell us what you've done."

"Thanks Eileen, and thank you, board members for inviting me. Poignant stories will be in our paper over the next few weeks. Several people Dr. Barrett referred to me have been casualties of practices that PharmaTruth has been working to expose. They were brave to talk about their experiences," Ruth said. "They've given me accounts of private suffering and even I, used to hearing heart-rending tales, was deeply touched. May I have the lights out and the screen down please."

Belsun moved around the room, resting her hands on the backs of the chairs of board members as she showed photographs of patients Hannah Dorst and Gwen Allen, summarizing their stories.

"Another courageous person volunteered to reveal his experiences with a pharmaceutical company. Dr. Norman Wise, a practicing physician, came clean about his dishonesty in pushing particular drugs in exchange for various favors, including money. Watch for the series in the *Register* and pay attention to feedback from readers and big Pharma."

The lights went back on, and Ruth turned the discussion back to Tom.

"So, the media blitz is on," he said. "A Publicity and Education Division, with composed talking points and a 'frequently asked questions' section have been added to the website. We're teaching volunteers how to respond to calls. For board members who'd like to learn more about this, call Laura Templeton and she'll arrange it. Thank you all for hanging in through these long meetings."

A deep sense of satisfaction, of making the right choice with his money and his life, flooded Tom as everyone filed out of the conference room. Unfortunately, it was followed by another feeling – one of trepidation. He knew firsthand that giants in power are not vanquished easily.

Chapter 30

Tom walked out of the meeting, smiled, gave thumbs up to those who caught his eye. But why was his stomach fluttering, and why had cold sweat formed on his head? He found George, his in-house confidant and therapist.

"George, after that terrific meeting why am I so nervous?"

"You don't know?" George said. "Sometimes I wonder, doctor, how you managed to pass all those tests in medical school. Okay, Ill fill you in. During the next few weeks, we're gonna be caught in a tsunami of attention. You'll be featured on radio and TV shows, some sympathetic, some critical. Pharma will call you names you've never heard of before. You'll get hate mail. I'll have to work harder to keep you safe. Get the picture?"

"Uh, well, yes, I guess. Wrestling with an octopus while drowning? Fair analogy?"

"Not that bad. It's gonna be challenging, but necessary. Bringing attention to this makes it easier for Rafferty and Brill. They'll get media coverage, and you know how politicians are addicted to that. So, my advice is to take some time now to relax, rest up, do some things that make you happy."

What makes me happy? Time with Cynthia.

"Hi, Cyn. I need a dose of you. Give me a call when you can."

That turned out to be the next day.

"Tom, sorry I haven't called back sooner, been busy as hell. What's up?"

"How 'bout a date tonight?"

"Damn, got a meeting tonight. How about tomorrow?" Negotiations for when and where commenced.

At three the next day, they met at the Worcester Art Museum to view an exhibition of Hudson River School artists. After wandering around for a couple of hours they went to Cynthia's condo. Tom told her how excited he was about PharmaTruth's progress.

"Sounds like you're really breaking through," Cynthia said. "By the way, have you heard anything from Barry about Katharine?"

Tom's eyes had been on an oil painting over the mantel but shifted to Cynthia. *Wonder why she has such a keen interest in a woman she'd never actually met, only saw her comatose in an Intensive Care Unit.*

"Nice of you to ask. I talked to her yesterday. She's starting rehab soon. But I'm worried. She sounded inappropriately euphoric. Didn't sound like the Katharine I knew."

He walked to the kitchen and poured a glass of wine, noticing a tremor in his hand as he spilled a few drops on the counter. He was struggling to understand his conflicted feelings about Katharine. And Barry. As he ruminated, his mood darkened.

"Losses pile up, more recent ones stoking up old embers I thought were cold," Tom said. "My dad used to tell me that sad events build character. I think that's bull. It's like an allergy. You meet up with a new loss and it triggers a memory response from your immune system. In allergies, you break out with a rash or have trouble breathing. With loss, I withdraw, go into my private space, hope the pain will go away and I can forget about it."

Cynthia moved behind Tom, wrapped her arms around him. "Let's call Barry and see how he's doing." Tom turned her around, gave her a hug. "Okay. Good idea."

"Barry, this is Tom Barrett."

"Tom, good to hear from you. How are you and Cynthia?

"We're fine. We're wondering about you and Katharine. What's happening?"

"She's in rehab and doing remarkably well. She's walking, talking, joking. Continuing to gain strength. The boys are still with Julie and Hunter Senior, getting along well in school. A big relief."

"Whew! I'm so pleased. Cynthia's here and wants to say hello." He put the phone on speaker.

"Hi Barry. Sounds like a lot of good news. When will she be going home?"

"Don't know yet. But it shouldn't be long now."

"How are you getting along?"

"I'm hangin' in there," he said in a tone that didn't sound like he was.

"Tell Katharine we called, and that we'll be calling her soon," Tom said. "Thanks for being the bearer of such good news. Let us know if there's anything we can do, okay? Talk to you soon."

"Speaking of health, what's the status of your hepatitis C?" Tom said, turning to Cynthia. This was a recurring discussion since Cynthia had told Tom of her positive test for hepatitis C. Being a nurse in an emergency room, where needle sticks were common, made her a prime candidate to contract this virus. It remained dormant in some people but could flare into outright hepatitis symptoms and lead to cirrhosis if not diagnosed and treated promptly.

"I'm embarrassed to say I've done nothing," she said. "My liver tests were initially slightly abnormal, but repeats reverted to normal," Cynthia said, looking down. "Everything I read about Hep-C is that your liver functions can be fine one day and a short time later go bad. My insurance won't cover the costs of the drug unless my liver function studies are abnormal. And even then, they won't cover most of the cost. And I have what's considered good coverage. It's like catch-22. I decided I can't afford to take the meds."

Tom tried to suppress a groan, but it slipped out. He had to restrain his paternalistic tendency to scold Cynthia like a recalcitrant child. Before he opened his mouth, he carefully considered his response, trying to fathom what prompts an insightful and knowledgeable health care professional to neglect her own wellbeing.

"You know, this is the kind of crap PharmaTruth is supposed to address. And here I am, the guy in charge of this wonderful do-good organization, dealing with a loved one who can't get meds because of cost," Tom fumed. "Tell me what kind of costs you're talking about."

"Well, taking a 12-week treatment regimen with two drugs costs around $150,000. There are others, but they're all super-expensive too. And depending on one's insurance coverage, out-of-pocket costs vary a lot, but they're all astronomical."

"So, here we are. You, the dean of a nursing school, with a good salary, good insurance coverage, at least in comparison to some others, and you feel you can't afford treatment for a disease that will kill you if left to run its course. That really sucks!"

"You won't get any argument from me. But what options do I have?"

"Well, I offered. What was it, four months ago, to pay whatever it cost to get the treatment for you, right?"

"I know. But I couldn't take the money at the time. We were breaking up, remember?"

"The offer is still good. In fact, if I can insist, I insist. Please."

"I'll talk to my gastroenterologist next week. I'm grateful, of course, that I have this option, but you know thousands of others who need the medication don't have such a good solution. What can PharmaTruth do about that?"

"Are you willing to testify at a congressional hearing about your experience?"

"What congressional hearing?"

Tom told her about Senator Rafferty and Representative Brill's plan for filing new legislation on drug costs and how there'd be hearings on the bills.

"Sure, I'd be glad to do that if you think it would do any good."

"It can't hurt. One never knows what comes out of hearings. But it's one way to get attention and maybe legislation to change this travesty. I'll add your name to a list of suggested witnesses for the hearings. In the meantime, please sign up for treatment. Please."

Tom leaned over, pulled Cynthia closer. "Can we go to bed now?"

Chapter 31

Warner strode around his office, agitated, like a stag in rut. He chain-smoked cigarettes, drinking straight bourbon, and barked at Shelby every time he came in.

"Shelby, find out where that bitch lives," he bellowed. "I want her so scared she'll do anything to get back into my good graces."

"Do you mind my asking what happened?" Shelby whispered.

"Yeah, I do mind. None of your fucking business. But I'll tell you one thing: she lost a once-in-a-lifetime opportunity to enjoy a great lifestyle once we get this drug out there and selling. Call the personnel department, get her home address. Another thing. Send her office computer to IT and have them sift through her emails and root through her office drawers, see if we can find something to threaten her with."

Shelby left, covertly shaking his head, suspecting what happened. Warner went to his window, looked at the river, plotted his next move. *I'll put a tail on her, scare her and see what that does. It's a shame. I liked her. Could have been fun in the sack.*

After he got Dina's address, Warner rented a non-descript car and found her house, a modest Cape Cod on Locust Street. He parked a few doors away, pulled out his iPad and tried to look busy as he waited, hoping to see Dina emerge from her house. Noon came with no action. He lost patience, went back to his office and called Shelby.

"Hire a detective to monitor her address," he told him. "I wanna know when she comes and goes. Uh, another thing. She has a daughter. Have the detective track her too."

***

George waited until darkness engulfed the leafy neighborhood around Dina's house to sneak in. She'd left her notes about Pylea in an envelope hidden in her clothes dryer when she and Debbie swept up their essential possessions. *Of all things to leave behind. Hell, it's probably my fault for hurrying them to leave.* He parked several houses away before heading for the driveway that led to the side door. Quickly, he unlocked the door, went to the laundry room, found the drier, retrieved the envelope. He left by the same door, hoping neighbors didn't notice this large Black guy slipping in and out of Dina's house in the dark.

The neighbors didn't notice. Warner's hired detective did.

Chapter 32

After dropping Dina off at her new place, George headed back to her old house. He used the side entrance again and stuffed the things Dina wanted into a shopping bag he found in the kitchen. He left by the same door. Glancing around, he didn't see anyone. Quickly, he walked down the street to his car and drove away.

Following him was a small, gaunt man in a black Toyota, the same guy who'd watched George yesterday. Maybe, he thought, this Black guy would lead him to the pay dirt he was after, where Dina Robbins was hiding out. Reginald Warner told him he'd pay him well to find where she'd gone.

George rang the doorbell at Dina's new house and waited. No response. *Why isn't she answering the door? I dropped her off not that long ago.* He called her.

"You okay?" he said.

"Yeah, I'm fine. Had to pick up Debbie at her friend's house. On my way home now."

"I left a package outside your front door. See you tomorrow."

"Thanks, George. Again."

The Toyota guy watched George leave and jotted down the address. He sat in his car to see if Dina came out to retrieve the shopping bag. About fifteen minutes later, a car arrived and parked in the driveway. Two women went inside.

He phoned Warner's number.

"This is Roy. I've found where she lives. 198 Knowles Drive, off Kensington. I saw her and a teenage girl come here and go inside. Her car is a red Honda 4-door, about eight years old, Mass license plate 599-WR2. Want me to do anything else tonight?"

"No, I got what I need. Don't want you for anything else. I'll send your money."

Warner rushed to his Ferrari and roared out of the garage, lighting a cigarette in the process. His GPS dictated the way. He pulled up a few yards from the front of her house on the opposite side of the street, and scanned the house and lot, plotting his next move.

Inside, Dina and Debbie were getting ready for bed.

"What are you doing tomorrow?" Debbie asked Dina. "Since you don't work at Pylea anymore, what do you do all day? Are you ever gonna tell me what happened? Did you get fired? Or just quit?"

"I'll stay busy, don't worry," Dina said. "I quit. I'll tell you all about it some other time. Not now, I'm tired. Goodnight, sweetie."

She wasn't ready to tell Debbie the truth about Pylea and that creep Warner. *She'd find out soon enough about malevolence. Let her keep whatever innocence she still had, as long as it might last.* She turned on her side and hoped she could sleep.

Warner quietly opened his car door, slid out from under the steering wheel, and eased the door closed. Scanning for people or sounds, he slipped past Dina's Honda. Warner sneered to himself that this was an ordinary blah suburban neighborhood where people were probably drinking beer, watching TV or playing computer games. At the porch stairs he hesitated and decided to go around to the back of the house, taking care not to trip over hidden obstacles on this overcast night. He reached what he assumed was a bedroom and stepped up on a rock in the side garden, peering inside. Nothing but darkness except for an illuminated clock on a table. He moved along the house wall to the next window and saw a young woman lying under covers using an iPad.

Must be her daughter, so that other bedroom must be hers. He went back and stared in again. Now that his eyes had become accustomed to the dark, he could see someone in bed. He leaned in to get a better look and lost his balance, falling with a loud thump against the exterior wall of the bedroom.

Next door a German Shepherd jumped off his bed and barked loudly, alarming anyone within a hundred yards. Dina rose in a panic, grabbed her phone, quickly called 911 first, then George.

Warner saw lights suddenly turned on in Dina's house and at the house next door where the barking dog had gotten more agitated. He froze, hearing the guttural bark of a dog he could tell was big. He had to get back to his car before anyone saw it. No one could mistake a red Ferrari that clearly didn't belong in this neighborhood.

He moved stealthily along the side of the house, hoping to elude detection by wary neighbors. The dog's owner opened his front door to see what was arousing his dog. His dog squeezed past him, sprinting down the lawn after Warner.

As he opened his car door, the dog caught up with him and massive German shepherd jaws clamped down on his ankle, sending searing pain up his leg.

"Goddammit, you sonuvabitch!" Warner screamed. Warner's kicks did nothing to dislodge the dog's hold on his ankle. He dropped onto the front seat, reached into the console and groped for his handgun. When he felt the cold steel, he slipped his forefinger around the trigger and swung around towards the dog. He fired directly at the animal's head.

The dog's owner, hearing the gunshot, abruptly stopped running toward his dog, incredulous and horror-stricken when he saw his precious dog slump onto the pavement.

Flashing blue lights flooded the street and sirens screamed as two police cruisers roared down the street. They skidded to the curb about fifteen yards to the right of Warner's car. Warner kicked the dog's carcass away, pulled his bleeding leg into his car and slammed his door shut. He spun his car around, hoping there was a way out to his left. His bloody foot floored the pedal, squealing rubber as the oversized motor surged, the car blazing away.

An officer jumped out of his cruiser at Dina's house, the other cop pursued Warner. He didn't have a chance. The cop radioed for help but knew a Ferrari had every advantage and would get away.

Dina and Debbie were frantic. Debbie had no clue what was happening, but Dina was sure who had provoked this melee. She'd already called George who was on his way. The neighbor whose dog had been killed talked to a policeman. His wife was crying and cradling the bloodied head of a lifeless dog in her lap in the middle of the street.

When George arrived, he rushed to Dina, and Debbie watched as George wrapped Dina in his arms. They turned and quickly included a confused and panicked Debbie in their embrace. They went inside with the policeman.

"May I say a few things?" George said.

"Who are you? What are you doing here?" one officer asked George, warily eying this large Black guy.

Dina jumped in. "George Logan; he's with me. I called him to come."

"Okay, what do you want to say?"

"Number one, I'm sure that guy who ran off is a man named Reginald Warner. I can go into how I'm sure of that later. Number two, if that big dog had his jawbone around Warner's leg, his wound's gotta be bad, and he'll need medical attention. Probably makes sense to alert local emergency rooms to look out for a guy with a dog bite on his ankle. Three, he parks his bright red Ferrari in a garage in Cambridge. Dina, you can tell them where that is. There's bound to be blood on the floor and door of that car."

"Yeah? How do you know this is the guy?"

"I used to work for him," Dina said. "Recently, he was totally inappropriate, and I quit. Suddenly. He's not the kind of person who can accept not having things go his own way. I've been in that car before."

"I see. Okay, write down his garage address and we can follow up tomorrow if we need further information.

After taking the paper from her, the officer looked at George before heading back to his squad car. "Thanks for your help. Good night," the officer said.

As he left, George mentally flogged himself. *Sure, I helped. Helped lead someone here from Dina's old house. That's how Warner knew where to find her.*

***

Warner's ankle was throbbing. Bleeding had stopped but his ankle had already ballooned and could hardly bear any weight. His head was woozy as he parked his car. He called Shelby and told him to come to the garage right away. When Shelby got there, Warner was nearly unconscious.

"Reggie!" Shelby shook him by the shoulders. No response. "Reggie!" He slapped his face a couple times.

Coming to, Warner told Shelby he'd been bitten by a vicious dog and asked Shelby to get him into his condo.

"Reggie, you gotta go to a hospital," Shelby said after looking at his bloody leg. Even as he said it, he knew Warner would refuse.

"Get me to my condo!" he screamed. "I only need to clean this ankle up, get a bandage on it and I'll be fine!"

Shelby, in his usual sheep-like fashion, obliged. In Warner's condo, he cleaned up the gruesome wound, nearly passing out as he looked at the shining tendon sheaths below the torn skin and muscle.

"Boss, this looks real bad. You need a doctor."

"I'm not goin' to an ER, stop nagging me. This'll get better on its own. I had a dog bite like this when I was a kid in Texas. My pappy wouldn't take me to a doctor, but I got better anyhow. That's what'll happen now."

"You're not a kid anymore, Reggie. Please let me take you."

"Get out! I'll take care of this myself. Go!"

Shelby skulked out, looking back at Warner, who was looking increasingly pale. But what could he do? He considered his options: leave and worry all night about his boss or slip into the other room and stay alert for any change. After an hour listening from the other room, Shelby heard Warner snoring. Shelby turned over on the couch, listening for any change in his boss's breathing pattern and hearing none, relaxed and fell asleep.

By morning, Warner had a high fever. In his delirium he'd knocked over the bedside water pitcher and was incontinent. He tried to get out of bed, but his ankle was so painful he groaned and rolled back.

Shelby woke up, startled by sounds emanating from Warner's bedroom. He rushed in. Warner was incoherent and writhing in bed. Shelby called 911 and within several minutes the emergency responders hustled Warner to Sparks Hospital in Cambridge.

"Horrible dog bite with infection," one of the doctors said to a nurse. "I've taken cultures, given him a tetanus booster and we're pushing broad spectrum antibiotics intravenously."

"What did he say about the bite?"

"He's completely out of it. Guy who brought him doesn't know squat about how or why he got bitten."

"I got word on the internet that local emergency rooms got an alert to watch out for a dog bite victim that happened under unusual circumstances" the ER Chief said when he came on duty. "Some guy was prowling around a woman's house and a neighbor's dog got loose and bit him. The guy pulled a gun and shot the dog dead! He got away but cops figure he'd show up in an ER. Maybe this is that guy."

"He killed a dog? I hate to treat people that despicable," one of the nurses complained.

"You know we have no choice. Let's get him up to surgery so they can debride the wound."

By the next morning his fever had risen to 105 degrees and stayed up all day. The following day on rounds, the resident told his team, "Bad news. They cultured meth-resistant staph aureus. This guy's in trouble." They pushed more intravenous antibiotics, but Warner's fever didn't budge. Shelby came to visit.

"You have to put on gown and gloves to go in there," the nurse admonished.

Shelby complied, his usual default for everything. He approached Warner's bed with trepidation, not knowing what to expect. What he saw stunned him. Warner was flushed with fever, his eyes glazed like wax, his movement minimal.

"Reggie, it's me, Shelby. Can you hear me? Can I do anything for you?"

Getting no response, Shelby lingered for a moment then turned to leave.

"Shelby," a growl came. "Is that you? Where am I?"

Shelby, startled to hear his boss's voice, spun on his heels and rushed back to his bedside.

"Reggie, it's me. How're you doin'?" He was oblivious to how incongruous his question was.

"Feel rotten. Get me outta here." He slumped back and fell asleep.

Shelby, in a most uncharacteristic act, stopped at the nurses' station.

"Pardon me, my name is Roy Shelby. I'm Mr. Warner's secretary and his friend. He's the head of Pylea Pharmaceuticals here in Cambridge. Our company has a drug specific for resistant infections and it seems that's what's wrong with Mr. Warner. Is there a chance I could talk to his doctor?"

The nurse looked at him skeptically.

"What is your name again? And where do you work?"

Shelby repeated what he'd said. "I could provide the drug to the hospital. It's been approved by the FDA, but our company hasn't released it yet."

The nurse stared at him briefly, then called her supervisor. After Shelby told the nursing supervisor the same thing, she called Dr. Rivkin, Warner's attending physician and returned to the nurses' station.

"Mr. Shelby, Dr. Rivkin would like to speak to you." Ten minutes later, Dr. Rivkin came, and Shelby reiterated what he'd told the nurses.

"Can you obtain this medication for us?"

"I'll talk to some people at the company and see what I can do," Shelby said.

Even Shelby was surprised at the speed with which Pylea got the drug to Sparks hospital. In short order, the drug and its delivery system were set up at Warner's bed and the infusion began.

Miraculously, a day later, his fever was down. He could sip apple juice and with help, sit up in bed. The doctors told him Cidal had been incredibly successful. Warner grinned, knowing this could only help promotion. He could see it now: "The owner himself was rescued from the throes of death by the drug his own company was manufacturing." He grinned to himself to think how shocked the hospital would be when they got the bill.

***

George went to the local police station, and they told him the assailant-- typical cop-talk-- got away in his Ferrari.

"Any local medical facilities report seeing a man with a dog bite?" he asked.

"Can't share that with you, partner. Sorry." George worried that if Warner was on the loose, he could come back, so he took Dina and her daughter to his place.

"Dina, until we know where Warner is, you and Deb need to stay here," he said. "At least I'll be around if he tries anything else. Can't believe I didn't consider someone following me. I'm supposed to be a great detective. More like Inspector Clouseau."

"C'mon George, don't be so hard on yourself. We feel safe here. But I feel bad about that poor dog and his owner. I didn't know those folks, but that dog was friendly," Dina said. "Sure was a good watchdog. Can you imagine what might have happened if that dog hadn't barked and gotten out?"

"No, he probably saved your life, or at least spared you an ugly confrontation with Warner," George said, looking directly at Dina. "I wonder where he is. Think this will be on TV news?"

It was. Neighbors were interviewed on camera, saying predictable things about how surprised they were that this happened on their quiet little street. Massachusetts Society for the Prevention of Cruelty to Animals issued a statement condemning the killing of the dog "horrendous."

George perked up when he heard police were interviewing a "person of interest" with a dog bite on his ankle, but they didn't identify him or the hospital.

"The logical assumption is that Warner went back to his condo and to a hospital nearby. I'm going to snoop around Cambridge hospitals. You and Debbie stay here. Phone me stat if you need me or hear anything."

George went to Mt. Auburn Hospital and asked at the Visitor's Desk where he could find Reginald Warner. A woman in her mid-seventies, clearly a volunteer, looked at her computer, shook her head, and told George there was no record of anyone by that name in their hospital. He thanked her, went to another hospital and got the same answer. His third stop was at Sparks Hospital where a volunteer at their visitor's desk said, "Yes, he's in room 760. Take one of those elevators over there to the 7th floor, turn left. Room 760 is a couple of doors down."

The volunteer looked at his computer again, and added, "Oh, wait a minute. Sorry. We have restrictions: he can have no visitors except one man who's his secretary." He looked up apologetically and said once more, "I'm very sorry."

George didn't want to visit him. He only wanted to know where he was. Now he knew what to do. He called his friend Collin, a private detective, and asked him if he could do a little work for him.

"What kind of work, George?" Collin asked.

"Surveillance." George told him about wanting Warner tailed when he got out of the hospital.

***

"It might be better to wait until tomorrow," the nurse told the two cops outside of Warner's hospital room. "I don't think he's completely with it yet."

"We'd sure like to talk to him today, if at all possible," one said.

"Let me check on his vitals, then I'll let you know."

The nurse came out after checking his blood pressure, pulse and temperature. He held the door open for them, gesturing them in. Even in his weakened state, Warner saw uniforms and knew policemen when he saw them. His face tightened.

"What is this? Why have you let cops in here?" Warner said, the corners of his mouth downturned.

"We want to ask you a couple of questions," one of officers said. "You remember being on Knowles Drive two nights ago?"

"Nah, never heard of a Knowles Drive," Warner replied. "What the hell is this about?"

"Remember being bitten by a German shepherd?"

"No." he said, looking them straight in the eyes. Warner had experience dealing with law enforcement.

"We have a couple of eyewitnesses who said a man fitting your description killed their dog."

"Huh? Killed their dog? What're they talkin' about?"

The cops recorded his denials and told Warner they'd be back to talk again in a day or two. "I'm not gonna be here much longer," Warner told the police as they were leaving.

"We know where to find you," one of them said.

Because George had told them where to look, they'd found his Ferrari in his parking space at the condo garage. After getting a search warrant, they took swabs of blood on the floormats and were in the process of matching this to blood samples taken from the dead German Shephard's mouth. They had their man but waited to make an arrest until all the evidence collection was completed.

Chapter 33

George wangled an appointment at the Massachusetts Attorney General's office to talk to a staff lawyer. In his hand were the transcribed version of Dina's notes about Warner and Pylea and David Longstreet's summary of her entire undercover operation. George was sure this would be a potent weapon as the Attorney General continued her probe of big pharma. But if it were made public it could put Dina in an even more precarious spot. Warner would inevitably discover where she'd moved, and George feared he might go to extreme measures to silence her.

"George Logan?" a young woman called out.

"Right here."

She approached George cautiously. With a sigh, she invited him into a small, windowless office. "Please take a seat. I'm Erin Finley." She knew little about why she was meeting George and her perfunctory attitude indicated she wasn't particularly interested and was impatient to get this over with.

George reeled out the Pylea story, slowly at first, and more urgently when he discussed Dina Robbin's role in gathering information and details of her experiences. Finley slipped on her reading glasses and took Longstreet's summary of Dina's conversations with Warner. As she read

George could tell her interest perked up after the first few sentences.

"This is extraordinary," she said, crossing and uncrossing her legs as she read. "I thought the Purdue case was an exception, that they were a rogue company. I still think they are, but this company and Warner are also breaking a bunch of laws," she said. "Can Dina come in and give a deposition? We need to begin working on this, to build a case."

"That's what I'm here to arrange. You tell me when, and we'll be here. It's gotta be soon because, as you can imagine, Dina's at risk," George said. "She's currently in an undisclosed location, but knowing Warner, he'll be in a no-holds-barred search mission. We're extremely concerned about her safety. She needs to get this on the record pronto, directly to you."

"Let me get that set up right now." She punched a number into her phone and within a few minutes had secured a time.

"How about tomorrow at two?"

"Done. That's great. Thanks for such a prompt response. Who said the government can't get anything done?"

"Some things take longer than others. You gotta realize, though, this is step one. A damned big one, but still, the rest takes longer. Maybe months."

The next day, Dina, George, and David Longstreet sat in folding chairs; a court reporter readied her equipment. Dina brushed stray strands of hair from her forehead, fidgeted with her belt, and tried to sit still in the cold metal chairs. After a few false starts, questioning commenced. Dina took several deep breaths, told her story in calm cadences and complete sentences. At 3:45 p.m. it was over. She knew this was only the first few yards of a marathon.

"We'll have to get documentation from Pylea, transcripts of emails, phone calls, minutes of meetings, all that," Erin told them. "Then we'll subpoena records from insurance companies that Warner allegedly bribed with stock. Those insurance execs had to know their companies couldn't receive stock shares from Warner. Company transactions are public and discoverable. If there is evidence of stock transfers, we'll discover it by how they directed stocks to be given to spouses and children, with or without their knowledge.

"Now, on to other issues. We'll track down and talk to doctors he's hired and hospital executives he's spoken with. Some of it we may never get or see. But this is a great start." She looked over their heads, lost in her legal world. "We're still dealing with fallout from the Purdue and Insys cases. It's almost like Jarndyce v. Jarndyce in Bleak House. Goes on forever. But this – this will take precedence over other cases."

***

"You did great, Dina," George said as they left One Ashburton Place.

"I agree," David said. "You were clear, concise, convincing. I'd use you as a witness in any case! See you guys later. I've got to get back to the office."

"I'm glad people who can do something listened. Maybe it'll do some good," Dina said. "George, you seem distracted. What's up?"

"How's Debbie adapting?" George asked, returning to a subject troubling him.

"She worries a lot, but she's looking forward to college, hoping classes will begin by September. These are good indicators she's adjusting."

"And you? Have you adjusted?" George asked.

"Well, like everyone, you get attached to your home. That reminds me, there are some more things at my house I'd appreciate you getting for me. Hate to ask you all the time to be my fetcher, but I don't know how else…"

"Tell me what you want, and I'm happy to get it," George interrupted. "No problem. Hey, it's almost dinnertime. Wanna join me at one of my favorite places? It's down off Charles Street. Wonderful, authentic Persian food, atmosphere is perfect. Quiet, with great Iranian art all around."

"Doubt I'd run into Warner there. He hates all things ethnic. I'd love to join you."

"Then after dinner, I'll get what you need from your house. Your car down here?"

Over their delicious, aromatic meal, Dina looked at George from a different perspective. She'd had inklings of attraction since she'd met him, but his recent caring and dedication had stirred emotions she hadn't felt for…how long? She wondered if he was even aware of her developing affection for him.

"George, tell me more about yourself. I feel so indebted to you for all you've done for me. After our first meeting when, I must admit, I was kind of pissed that Tom sprung you on me. I was struck by your, what should I call it, understanding of people? How'd you get that way? I don't know if I've ever heard you talk about yourself."

"My least favorite topic of conversation," he said with a wry smile. "Actually, I've led a fairly boring life." He had told her before about his boyhood, his folks, and now he added a miniscule summary of his war experiences, how he'd met Tom and their adventures.

"Never married?"

"Nope."

"Gay?"

When he stopped laughing, he said, "Nope again. Just haven't found the right woman."

"What are you looking for in the *right* woman?"

"Ha, I'm not looking for her," he said, looking away.

"C'mon, George, give me a break. You're not some cold fish with zero feelings. You must have fantasies about the ideal woman."

"Well, as they say about other things, 'I'll know it when I see it.'"

Dina glanced down at her plate, poked at some abandoned scraps of food. Should she take this conversation a step further?

"What do you see when you look at me?"

He gazed at her intently, trying to decide how to respond. Measuring his words, he said, almost inaudibly, "I see a very attractive, intelligent, and caring woman. I see someone committed to a cause, who's courageous. I see someone I care about."

"As I look at you, I see someone I care about too." She reached her hand across the table, placing it on his. "I'd be interested in getting to know each other outside of your assignment to protect me. Is that possible?"

George was aware of a pulsation in his head, a flushing sensation in his face. He took a deep breath.

"Lordy, lordy, as my mother used to say when she was astounded by a twist in reality. I'm....I don't know what I am. Surprised, I guess. Answering your question: yes, I'd like to get to know you better. But are you sure you know what you'd be getting into? You remember I have PTSD? That I'm Black and you're not? And your daughter hates me?" He chuckled as he said that.

"She doesn't hate you. She likes you." Dina's words came like boulders tumbling down a cliff. "Those other things you mentioned. Neither of us can do a damned thing about them. Your post-traumatic stress seems to be under control. Is it?"

"I feel better now than I've felt for many months. It may be the medication, it could be I have a purpose in life, or whatever. Will my PTSD stay under control? Neither I nor my doctors can say. But I feel good about the prospects."

"About the Black thing: the world's different than it was, even ten years ago. Mixed race couples are much more common," Dina said.

A grin stole across George's face.

"You didn't grow up where I did. Things have changed...to some degree," he said. "A lot of people thought Obama's presidency would change everything. I thought he was the ideal kind of man to bring about attitudinal change. To some extent he did. But implicit bias still exists even in good people who may be trying hard to change. But the culture you grow up in sears beliefs into your mind. These aren't easily reshaped. I feel it every day. I'm a big fellow, and white people eye me cautiously, thinking that at any moment I'll become a threat."

"Honestly, I never thought about how that would feel, having people automatically assume the worst about you like that," Dina said. "I'm probably guilty of it too, to some extent, I'm ashamed to say. It must be so hard and disappointing to live with this constantly."

George looked into Dina's eyes. *Could this work? At least she's not being defensive.*

The waitress sidled over to their table, offering a dessert menu. They both demurred, apologizing for rejecting the temptations. They ordered tea.

George pushed back from the table, crossed his legs, folded his hands in his lap. *Now what?*

"I'm sorry if I'm coming on too strong," Dina said. "Maybe I need to slow down a little bit. Maybe I'm feeling vulnerable and romanticizing you as my savior. But I do have feelings for you and hoped you might also."

"I do. I've pushed my feelings aside because of all that stuff I just talked about," he said. "Let's get you out of this Warner mess and then sort this out. Okay?"

Dina knew he was right. She looked down at her teacup, sighed and said, "Okay. But after this is past, promise me that you'll allow yourself to explore these feelings."

George smiled, took her hands in his, kissed them, and gave her a wink.

Chapter 34

Tom was swept up in a blur of PharmaTruth disclosures, reported in depth by Ruth Belsun, unleashing a cyclone of contentious charges. The pharmaceutical industry wasn't blind or deaf to this swirl of media, prompting consumer and political attention. They furiously mobilized counterattacks, relying on massive advertising campaigns rationalizing their high prices by claiming monumental expenses for research and development of new wonder drugs. In their media blitz they urged consumers to appreciate they'd created incalculable numbers of remedies for diseases of humankind.

Which was true. Tom, in moments of deep reflection, marveled at what a mixed bag pharma was. Most companies were populated by hundreds of hard-working, dedicated scientists, businessmen and women, and lawyers sorting through and trying to make sense of a maze of laws and regulations in a crazy quilt called pharma. With these conflicting thoughts obsessing him and keeping him awake, he recognized he needed a break.

"Cyn, how about a date? Soon? Gimme a call," he texted.

"Just thinking of you in this lovely weather. How about this weekend? Go somewhere warmer than here?" she texted back.

"We could resurrect that Bahamas trip we scrubbed when we went to San Diego to see Katharine. Call me so we can have an audible conversation!"

They settled on Nassau where the forecast was sunny, in the mid-seventies. After a short flight from Boston, they checked into the Rosemont Hotel, Saturday at noon. After lunch they strolled on the beach, had several pina coladas, then returned to their room and made love.

When they woke from a light slumber, lolling about in bed, Cynthia rolled toward Tom. He thought she was tempting him again. He kissed her neck, and as he did, she surprised him by asking, "Have you heard anything from Katharine?"

Confused that she would ask about Katharine right after they'd made love, he replied, "As a matter of fact, yes. What in hell made you think of her? Are you jealous, or what?" he teased.

"Of course. She's a lovely young woman and you're an attractive single man. And I love you, you lunkhead. Why shouldn't I be jealous?"

Tom looked at Cynthia and kissed her again.

"She emailed me. She has a new man in her life, a guy named Jordan, so you can forget about being jealous. Told me all about it. I think she wanted my blessing. God knows why."

"Oh? Not Barry?"

"No, Barry's a nice guy but I never thought he was number one for her. I feel bad for him. I think he truly loved her and stood by her through her hospitalization. But things happen. And perhaps her personality change was part of it.

"You know, my relationship with her is odd. In a way, I feel responsible for her, which I know is ridiculous, but she was Danny's wife, and I guess I transferred my affection for him to her."

"Were you in love with her?" Cynthia asked, in her straight-from-the-shoulder way.

"Uh, let's see. The hackneyed answer is 'I loved her, but I was not in love with her.' I don't know," he stammered, "I was physically attracted to her, but I had the feeling that it wouldn't work out. To me there was always a sense of disloyalty to Danny if I got involved with his wife, even though he was dead, for chrissakes. Almost like cheating on your best friend," he said. "Isn't that weird?"

"Not weird. It's curious how personal loyalties shape our actions. Most people, I'd say, wouldn't let that sort of thing get in the way of their own happiness. It speaks volumes about your Eagle Scout morality, your sappy Calvinism. Still, it's one of your more endearing qualities.

"Who's the lucky guy she's with, this fellow named Jordan?" Cynthia said.

"Well, not surprisingly, he's a surgeon, like Danny and me. He was on the team caring for her head injury. Katharine must have a thing about surgeons," he laughed. "They started seeing each other while she was in rehab. It took off like a zephyr, according to her. Who knows, we might get invited to their wedding."

Tom's phone rang. He scrambled out of bed and fumbled through his clothes to retrieve it.

"George! What's up?"

George, speaking rapidly, told him about Warner's prowling debacle and how he landed in the hospital with the infected dog bite.

"Cops put the pieces together and are charging him with destruction of property, to wit, a dog he killed, stalking, trespassing, leaving the scene of a crime, resisting arrest, and maybe other things. They found his DNA on a broken shingle on the back wall of Dina's house, apparently smudged there when he tripped and broke his fall with his hand. They matched it with DNA from blood in his car."

"I didn't know about any of this," Tom said.

"That's why I called. It's all over the local TV and news media. On top of that, the Attorney General has filed suit against him detailing shenanigans with Cidal, how Pylea is price-gouging, making illegal deals with insurance companies, a few other things. The suit goes on and on," George said, slowing down to his normal pace of speech. "Dina's notes are key in this and coupled with recovery of his private phone and emails by subpoena, are gonna sink this bastard. I hope. But you never know with trials. Seems the bad guys know how to slither away from guilty verdicts. Especially the rich ones with expensive lawyers."

"Are you keeping Dina safe through this? Any goons lurking about?"

"She and Debbie -- you know, her daughter -- are at my place. I don't know if she should go back to either her home or the so-called safe house, safe until dumb me led Warner's detective there. Any suggestions?"

"Find a new place, as inconvenient as that is. We've got to ensure Dina and her daughter stay safe. Is Warner free to move about?"

"He's out on bail, so yes, whatever his twisted psyche impels him to do is possible. I have a tail on him, but he could, and probably does, have agents I don't know about."

"I think we have to move Dina and Debbie out of the Boston area."

"Oh God, Debbie's a high school senior. Worst time in the world to move. She'd have to leave all her friends and graduate from an unfamiliar school she's never taken a class in."

"Could she live with one of her friend's families until she graduates? She's not the target, Dina is."

"I worry she could be taken as hostage. Know that sounds dramatic, but Warner is a snake. I'll talk to Dina and Debbie about this. For now, they're safe with me."

"Call me after that conversation. I'm in Nassau with Cynthia and we were having a great time until you called. Thanks, George," he said, teasing his friend. "We'll be home tomorrow night."

"Always glad to be of service, boss," George said. "I'll call you later. Say hello to Cynthia. The three of us need to get together again. It's been a long time, maybe since we were at Zylinski, that I've even seen her."

***

"Dina, we need to talk," George said. "Tom has some thoughts. When will Debbie be back?"

"About a half hour. She's at soccer practice. So, what's the talk about, as if I didn't know?"

"Tom thinks we need to move you again. I told him how difficult that would be, considering Deb is in her last year of high school. But Warner is a spiteful, vindictive wild card, and he's made bail. Protecting the two of you is top priority. Any ideas?"

Dina clenched her fists, and her face collapsed.

"Enough is enough," she screamed as long-suppressed tears gushed from her eyes. "How much do I have to take?

I should never have gotten myself into this. My great impulse to save the world! What crap! The world sucks, people suck. Why should I care? Mom's dead, one of the last good people on earth. All I wanted was to help get a drug out that would kill resistant organisms, and this is what I get for that? It's not gonna bring Mom back. And now I'm supposed to deny my daughter her high school graduation with the kids she's grown up with? No, I won't do that! Never!"

George wisely kept silent. *She has every right to be angry.* He waited, didn't put his arm around her for fear of being pushed away. The sun moved out of a break in the clouds and lit up the room, dust particles danced about in the air.

"Tom wondered if Debbie might move in with a friend's family to finish school and graduate with her friends. Is that a possibility?"

"I don't know. I really don't. This whole business is so disgusting. When she gets home, she and I will have to talk it out. Let me first talk to her alone. Contrary to what you worry about, she likes you. But I think I need to discuss options with her by ourselves."

"Of course. I'll take my lead from you. When she gets here, I'll disappear into my room. You call me out when the time's right."

When Debbie came back from soccer, Dina presented her with this unpleasant news. She took it like a root canal. George heard crying, yelling, then things being slammed down. George hoped none of them were valuable. They were so loud, he heard Debbie blaming her mother for getting them into this. Dina defended her actions, claiming it was her moral obligation to expose gross injustice, an argument that Debbie wasn't buying. Angry accusations, punctuated by sobs, subsided after both had worn out their rage. Debbie grudgingly recognized her dependence on her mother and Dina acknowledged her love for her daughter.

They tapped on George's closed door. Two exhausted and downcast, red-eyed women stared at the floor in front of them. They all stood stock-still, waiting for someone else to speak; it felt like minutes crept by in awkward silence.

"We'll get through this only by keeping our cool," George began, knowing Debbie could resent whatever he said. "Debbie, I know you feel you've been treated unfairly since you had nothing to do with this predicament. I agree with you, it's not fair. But your mother and I do want what's best for you, despite appearances. What we need to figure out is how. You have any ideas that might help us?"

Debbie looked at George, bewildered by her sense of being suspended in space, with nothing solid to hold onto.

"I don't want to lose my friends," Debbie said with tears again streaking down her cheeks. "I want to graduate with them like a normal kid, not some freak who has to move around like some kind of fugitive. I've moved too many times since Mom and Dad split and I'm sick of it."

George nodded with sympathy showing in his eyes.

"Who's your best friend?" George asked.

"Sue Collins, I guess."

"Dina, do you know her parents?"

"Vaguely. I've talked to her mother at a couple of PTO meetings."

"Debbie, have you been to her house?'

"Oh yeah, lots of times. Why?"

"You think her parents would let you live there until we get this thing sorted out?"

"I have no idea."

"I'll call her mother," Dina said. "The worst she can say is no."

***

Tom and Cynthia got home late Sunday night and crawled into bed at Tom's place. Just as they were falling asleep, Tom's phone buzzed.

"Shit. Only person I know calling me at this hour is George." Looking at his phone, he said "Yup, it's George."

"Hey. We're home, just got in bed," Tom said.

"Just letting you know, Dina's staying with me and Deb's moving in with her friend Sue's family until she graduates. The Collins family was terrific, very understanding. Restores my faith in people," George said. "We'll pack Deb's things and get UPS to pick them up and deliver them. Same thing with Dina's belongings, we'll ship them UPS here to my place. I called the AG, and they never got back to me, so we didn't want to wait to get them both settled."

"So how was your time away?"

"Great, had a wonderful but too short time. We'll go back there, maybe on our honeymoon."

"Your what?"

"You heard me. We're getting married. We decided in Nassau. How 'bout that?"

"Congratulations! That's so great! I'm happy for you both," George said.

"When's the big day?"

"To be determined. We have to work the details out; you know, church wedding or civil, in Boston or at some destination, all that kind of stuff," Tom said. "Wanna talk to Cyn?"

"Cynthia, that news makes my day. My best to you. I always hoped you'd do this. I'm at a loss for words."

"We're both finally at peace. It's been a long slog, but we know it's the right thing to do. Thanks for your blessing. That means a lot to us."

After the call George sat quietly, his thoughts a jumble of emotions -- happiness for his friends, his own sense of loneliness, confusion about his relationship with Dina, and uneasiness about what would happen next with Warner and his henchmen. His eyes closed as darkness crowded out daylight and within minutes, he was asleep in his chair.

Chapter 35

"Tom, Ruth Belsun here. Have you heard the news?"

"Hi Ruth. What news?"

"Wuhan, a city in China, has a big problem with a virus. It's called a 'coronavirus' and it's spreading like wildfire. Their government quarantined the whole damned city -- 11 million people. And the authorities are expected to lock down the whole Hubei Province, nearly 60 million people."

"Holy shit! Where'd the virus come from?"

"The scientists say it's a mutation from an animal virus now infecting humans. They call it a 'novel' virus. They've named the disease SARS-CoV2 since it's a respiratory illness like that SARS outbreak a few years ago. The World Health Organization is warning this is going to spread all over."

"How do they know what it is?"

"They take nasal swabs and can identify the RNA that's characteristic for this virus."

"Any treatment?" Tom realized how far away from clinical medicine he'd drifted.

"Not yet. They're trying out some things, but nothing seems to touch it. They say fatality rate is low, but there are so many cases the number of deaths will be high."

"Ruth, thanks for letting me know. That's horrible. Shades of Ebola. I'm sure the CDC or World Health

Organization will issue protocols for us to follow. Is this being covered by television stations?"

"They're all over it, yes. The president has been saying that it's all 'under control and it'll work out well,' in his words. I guess he's listening to his preferred TV station rather than scientists who say this could be devastating. Epidemiologists predict it could affect health care systems in every community, national and global economies and, closer to home, your efforts to get Congress to pay any attention to any legislation not aimed at dealing with this virus. That means problems in the pharma industry would go on the back burner."

"Thanks for the alert," Tom said. A flood of thoughts swept over him about losing momentum. "I'll talk to some of my infectious disease friends to get their take on this."

He opened his news links and read more. "We have it totally under control," Trump boasted in a hastily called news conference. *He'll surely get experts together to manage this threat for the United States.*

On January 30th, Leonhardt wrote in the New York Times that "the World Health Organization declared coronavirus to be a 'public-health emergency of international concern.' It announced 7,818 confirmed cases around the world." At the same time Trump assured the country that "We think we have it very well under control." Tom called Mike Berman with rising concern.

"Mike, I'm calling to get your opinion about this coronavirus outbreak. The President keeps saying it's only a flu and we don't have a problem in this country. What do you think?"

"He's full of shit, as usual. He's ignoring scientific information and his own medical advisors. This could be a major plague and he's acting like it's the common cold."

"What do you think we can do about it?"

"Unfortunately, nothing. Until the president stops listening to his preferred source of news and starts paying attention to scientists, he's going to lead us off a cliff."

Tom stared out his window. *People's rising crescendo of interest in limiting Pharma's strangle hold on drug prices will be dwarfed during a pandemic wrecking our society. I hope that Trump is right, for once, about this being contained.*

Over the following days, the President continued to give reassurances that everything was "going to be fine" and "we're in very good shape," painting a rosy picture of the Administration's policies about the virus. Tom was more worried by the day as he watched the president deny there was or would be a coronavirus problem. Health advisors from every sector were increasingly uncomfortable. Tom called Mike Berman again.

"I know why you're calling," Mike said. "Don't get me started about the president. He's managing this threat to the country in the worst possible way. He uses his typical simple-minded logic to downplay what could become the worst pandemic the world has seen since 1918. His supporters swallow everything he says and go on their merry ways, gathering together with each other, spreading the virus. I'm at my wit's end trying to figure out why people deny, deny, deny the threat when facts point in the exact opposite direction."

In time the stock market was reflecting the anxiety and over the next weeks it had plunged to levels that alarmed everyone. New York City was an epicenter of COVID-19 cases.

There was open disagreement by numerous governors with the president about the need for ventilators and other protective equipment for health care workers. Other governors were having their own problems with the president who complained about the "whiners" who should "get their own supplies." Most states were in quarantine mode with stay-at-home orders advised or even decreed. Daily state and local briefings outlined how citizens should protect themselves and others from viral spread.

PharmaTruth continued to collect data on corruption and helped to make the case against Warner as airtight as possible, switching to Zoom meetings while staff and volunteers worked from home. Tom watched, with trepidation, the burgeoning focus on the modern-day plague.

Nothing is simple. Just when I thought we were getting our act together to do something important for the health of the country, a pandemic arrives.

Other disconcerting news was that nearly half of the population had convinced themselves that the president was doing a good job despite his long delay in acting and surging numbers of cases and deaths. Congress passed a two trillion-dollar CARES bill to distribute money to people, small businesses and other entities, to prop up a failing economy.

The word from the Administration was that this onslaught of disease could continue through April, maybe May, or even longer. The scientists were finally able to convince the president that this scourge was serious and potentially calamitous. That it could threaten his re-election was the most likely argument to explain his turnaround. But even as the numbers of cases and deaths rose, he kept arguing that we needed to "open the country" and bring business back to life.

Case numbers and deaths continued to rise during the Spring and Summer. The stock market was like a roller coaster, one day rallying, the next spiraling downward. Disagreement over the course of action continued along politically partisan lines.

Conservatives worried more about the economy than the surge in cases and deaths, most other people feared the pandemic's impact on vulnerable populations and adhered to social distancing and the wearing of protective masks. Pundits and politicians could not predict the outcome of the November elections. Tom feared the worst: if the progressives didn't gain enough seats in both the House and Senate the Brill-Rafferty bill was dead on arrival.

Chapter 36

The terrain settled after a political earthquake had produced victory for progressives in the national elections. No one had been sure that a landslide in the house and senate, let alone the presidency, would come about.

Europe exhaled in relief, Asia recalibrated, Russia frowned, and a weary world hoped that long-standing dysfunctions in America's Congress would be mitigated. Legislators would at last address international issues lying in paralysis. The coronavirus pandemic was finally being addressed by most governors, and the pharmaceutical industry had worked furiously to develop treatment modalities for the virus and were closer to development and deployment of an effective vaccine.

Never one to let a critical moment slip past without quick response, Senator Rafferty called Eva Brill, who had narrowly won re-election.

"Eva, I'd say I was sorry about your party's fate, but that would be a lie. I'm delighted, of course, about the outcome. I hope you and I can still show what true bipartisan cooperation can look like. Can we huddle soon about crafting those companion bills about reining in pharmaceutical companies?"

"Well, we took a beating, that's for sure. I survived because of my district's hundred-year history of party loyalty regardless of nominee," she said. "I welcome the opportunity to work with you. We never were that far apart in our thinking on any number of issues. It's clear we need to do something about drug costs. I'm concerned that when a COVID-19 vaccine is released, the world will be at the mercy of whichever company reaches the finish line first.

"How should we begin? I'd like to get my mind off the election, so the sooner the better for me."

"How about tomorrow morning? My office at 10?" Senator Rafferty proposed.

"Perfect. See you then. I'll bring a staffer."

In contrast to Rafferty's and Brill's camaraderie, the rest of Washington was in an uproar. The changing of the guard was not a pleasant exercise in many quarters. Old tensions and blood feuds resulted in near physical confrontations as new lawmakers claimed their offices and departing legislators dragged their heels packing their wares and vacating space some of them had occupied for years. By day's end, many departing politicians were still up to their hips in boxes, empty liquor bottles strewn about as they growled at anyone who wandered into their space.

Since Rafferty had four more years in his term as senator, his office was calm, his staff unchanged. They were prepared with coffee and tea, pastries and bagels, when Brill and her aides arrived. As was the case everywhere now, everyone wore masks, and social distancing was the norm.

"Going over notes from our meetings at PharmaTruth and from constituents' concerns, here are things I think legislation should address," Rafferty said as he passed a ten-item list to the group. "We need to winnow this down to doable measures and draft a bill. The two committees I foresee having hearings for this in the Senate are Finance, which deals with Medicare; and Health, Education, Labor and Pensions (HELP) a big umbrella committee under whose aegis is the Federal Drug Administration (FDA), Centers for Disease Control and Prevention (CDC), National Institutes of Health (NIH), Substance Abuse, Mental Health, and Aging. The progressive majority now holds chairs of both committees, so for the first time in years we have a chance to do something significant."

"However," Congresswoman Brill said, "there is still a worrisome number of politicians whose pockets have been lined with pharma-lobby money. Hopefully constituent pressure will pull enough of them over to our side."

"We'll also need to do a little jawboning to persuade them it's in their best interests," Rafferty said. "I think the house and senate bills should:

- Require Medicare, Medicaid, the Veterans Administration, the Defense Department, and other federal government agencies that buy drugs to negotiate drug prices with pharmaceutical companies.
- Authorize regulations that cap out-of-pocket spending for copays on Medicare-prescribed drugs.
- Allow importation of drugs from other countries and make them available by prescription.
- Increase availability of generic drugs, shortening time that patents protect drugs from competition.
- Renew patents on existing drugs only when substantial changes have been made.
- Restore statutes that restrict direct advertising of drugs to consumers.

- Establish a statute making it a criminal offense to hire doctors to advocate for particular brand-name drugs.
- Regulate in-house drug research to require publication of all results, positive and negative.
- Place NIH monitoring scientists in pharmaceutical company laboratories."

"Some of these will fall away in committees and the House version may have some variation, which my staff is working on," Congresswoman Brill said. "But both will have basic areas of commonality."

Silence hung over the room as they studied the proposed legislation.

"Keep your wild applause down, please," Senator Rafferty said with his characteristic grin. "I know each of these will be met with resistance, even derision. And opposition will claim they're unconstitutional. I'm sure many, if not all, will be challenged in court if they become law. That's why we have this process called lawmaking."

Their staffs studied the list as they listened to his sonorous voice with a mixture of excitement and terror. This was going to be an overwhelming basketful of hard work. It was clear from Rafferty's demeanor that he wanted a quick turnaround on this sausage-making assignment.

"I expect chairs of both committees will heed our advice to invite consumers to testify. They'll ask pharma executives to offer their opinions. Opposition will be vociferous in condemning this bill as government interference in normal business activities, accusations of socialism and worse, but our recent electoral success suggests their voices will be less persuasive than they were under Mr. Twitter."

Brill looked down at her hands as Rafferty said this. Brill sincerely hoped these bills, whatever their final form might be, would curb runaway costs of essential medications.

"We have to craft an almost perfect bill," Rafferty went on. "Avoid downstream problems with implementation as there were in Obamacare. It must be designed to survive legal challenges."

Turning to both staffs, whose job it was to craft the language of the bill, Rafferty said, "You have a heavy responsibility to make this a law with watershed implications. I urge you to use every resource of our two offices. We'll both be looking for as many co-sponsors as we can persuade to join us. If any of you have connections to staff of new reps or senators, seek them out and get them to persuade their bosses to sign on.

"Some of you were with us at PharmaTruth's board meeting. You heard board members speak with deep knowledge and expertise. Continue to work with them. They want you to. Find other advisors. You know where to look, but fact-check anything you're told three times. Best of luck!"

"Thank you, Senator Rafferty," Congresswoman Brill said. "And I speak for my entire team when I say that it's exciting to usher in a new phase of bipartisan cooperation to help all Americans. I can tell you from personal family experience that drug costs must be contained. My daughter's family has a hard time keeping up. Her daughter has epilepsy and over the years has required several changes in her anticonvulsants. Each time they change, the cost of the new drug is much higher than her old drug. So, for me this is personal."

She didn't feel the need to add anything else to Rafferty's message. She wondered which moderate congresspersons in her party she could get to sign on to this.

Rafferty had a more formidable task, using his considerable powers of persuasion to nudge some of his opposite party colleagues to join him. He knew who he could work on but was unsure they'd go against their leadership. To do so would mean going against their big Pharma contributors and the silent but understood mission to maintain the way they conducted business.

Chapter 37

Ohio Congresswoman Brill was a seven-term Republican representative from Cleveland, a city consistent in electing moderate, sometimes liberal, congressmen and women. Brill was squarely a middle-of-the-road woman on social issues and leaned right on economic ones. She had a loyal following because of her careful attention to the needs of her constituents.

In this matter she and her staff felt ambivalent about Rafferty's nine items, some seemed too liberal. Worse, if Brill supported those measures and they became law, taking those positions would ensure she would never receive pharmaceutical company contributions for her future re-election campaigns. Her staff argued into the night but ultimately agreed they could sell the first seven in Brill's district. The last two -- regulating in-house research and having NIH monitors in company labs -- were too much, and they rejected those in fashioning the house bill. Facing election every twenty-four months, house members were in a constant state of fret with a wet finger in the air to figure out which way political winds were blowing. What new special interest group would grab headlines and influence voters?

Rafferty and Brill's staff persons fashioned identical companion bills to be introduced simultaneously in the house and senate. This bill made both left and right politicians equally unhappy, so it was considered a good compromise. Everyone wanted to get this done before recess.

Into the house hopper went the bill HR 2164, snaking its way through the pathway all bills take before reaching committee. In the house ways and means committee, it landed on Representative Becker's desk as chair of the subcommittee overseeing drug pricing. He presided over hearings with witnesses from advocacy groups, including PharmaTruth. After hearings it was reported out to the full house and passed with a comfortable margin. Now it was on to the senate.

Christian Blake, Democrat from Illinois, chaired the senate finance committee. The first witnesses he planned calling were consumers with complaints about drug pricing and availability. Executives from pharmaceutical companies would be next. Finally, he would get personnel from the federal agencies required to implement the elements of this proposed legislation.

"Welcome to the senate finance committee's hearing on the companion bills HR-2164 and S-247, entitled: An Act to Make Needed Prescribed Drugs Less Expensive and More Available, hereinafter referred to as the Brill-Rafferty Affordable Drugs Act."

Senator Blake laid out rules for the hearings, introduced committee members and called the first witness, setting a brisk tone for an efficient session.

"Hannah Dorst" the clerk sang out.

Hannah struggled to her feet, grasped handles on her walker, steadied herself and stood upright for a moment, making sure of her balance. Slowly, slowly she inched her way to the witness table, even though she was only settled in a seat two rows back. Casey Andrews helped ease her into a chair. He folded her walker and put it alongside the witness table. She looked up at Casey with a smile and he put his fingers to his lips in a kiss before returning to his seat. He was only a few feet from her in case she needed him. Casey knew how nervous Hannah was and had assured her he wouldn't be far away.

"Welcome Ms. Dorst," Senator Blake said, "and thank you for coming today. Any time during your testimony please tell me if you need anything. There's water there in front of you. Also, tell me if you need a break during your time with us."

Blake swore Hannah into the hearing.

"Thank you, Senator Blake," Hannah said strongly. "I'm a bit nervous, so bear with me if I'm a little slow to answer."

"Ms. Dorst, please tell us why you felt it necessary to make the trip to Washington. It mustn't have been easy for you," Blake smiled.

"When I was teaching, I always told my students that if they didn't speak up for themselves, nobody else would. I'm taking my own advice."

"You were a teacher?"

"Yes, both my husband, may he rest in peace, and I were elementary school teachers, back in the day."

Senator Blake looked down his list of committee members.

"Senator Rafferty, I believe Ms. Dorst is from your state of Massachusetts. Would you like to ask her some questions?"

"Thank you, Senator Blake. Ms. Dorst, add my thanks to Senator Blake's for coming today. Without invading your privacy, can you tell us about your medical condition? And what medicines you're taking?"

"Senator, you can take one look at me without invading my privacy and know I have arthritis. It's called rheumatoid arthritis, and I've been taking Humira for several years. It's very good for my arthritis. Problem is, it's getting so expensive I can't manage. So, I skip doses. That means more pain, more trouble getting around."

"Do you have insurance?"

"Yes, but it doesn't cover the whole cost. I have a co-pay that keeps getting higher and higher. I'm sixty-one years old. My teacher's pension health insurance isn't great, but I can't afford anything else. Who'd insure me with what I have? When I started taking Humira what I had to pay out of my purse was something like $1200. Now it's so much more I can't afford it. I have to go without it."

Senator Martz from Missouri followed Senator Rafferty. After a perfunctory thanking of Hannah for coming, he pulled his microphone closer.

"Ms. Dorst, have you ever taken advantage of any of the manufacturer's programs to help people in need?"

"I've tried almost all of them. Companies say over and over they have these special plans to help people with money problems, but, really, there are so many catches," Hannah said. "I always fall outside their guidelines 'cause my crummy little pension gives me more money than their rules allow.

"And it takes forever to apply for these things. The forms are, I don't know, I can't figure them out. They want me to send my income tax forms and prove I don't have savings and I'm not cheating. Even if I get what they say is available, copays are so high I couldn't afford them anyway.

I'm left to go with cheaper medicines that don't work nearly as well."

"What about the nurse ambassador program?" Martz said.

"That also depends on your insurance. If your insurance doesn't cover them, they won't come."

Senator Martz decided her answers were not shedding a good light on drug companies, a major source of his campaign war chest, so he yielded.

No other committee members asked for time, sensing Hannah's answers would not change the essence of her testimony.

"Anything to add Ms. Dorst?" Blake asked.

"Only to thank you for paying attention to this problem," she said, looking up at Senator Blake, gaining encouragement from his benign countenance. "You know, I'm not alone with this trouble paying for medicines. Friends tell me they've seen people crying at the drugstore when they hear how much their prescriptions cost. A lot of them, I heard, just walk away, leaving them on the counter. I hope you can do something about this. This shouldn't be happening in our wonderful country."

"Thank you again, Ms. Dorst," Blake said. "I hope your trip home is a pleasant one."

Casey stood and unfolded Hannah's walker, helped her up and positioned her in the frame. He gave her a little hug as they walked together out of the hearing room.

***

After a recess, Senator Blake called Barbara Simon to the witness table and swore her in. Simon was a large woman with hair the color of wheat. She moved with a lightness learned as a ballet student in her youth. An assertive woman who expected respectful attention when she spoke, she seemed at home in this august hearing room, a different sort of witness from Hannah Dorst, every senator's third grade teacher. After welcoming her, Blake called on Senator Shank from Utah.

"Ms. Simon, please tell us why you're here."

"Very simply, because I'm angry by the constantly rising price of insulin," she said in a strong voice. "I've been taking it for Type 1 diabetes since I was ten. That's twenty years now. The price has gone up 1000% since I started. That's a whole lot more than inflation of everything else. I have good insurance. I'm a librarian at the Brookline Public Library, but my monthly out-of-pocket cost for my insulin is nearly $1,000."

"The pharmaceutical industry is trying to help defray that cost, you know," Senator Shank said. "There are manufacturers' coupons to help people like you. Did you know that?"

"Of course, I know that" she said, responding sharply to his condescending tone. "I use those coupons, and my cost is still a thousand bucks every month. Figure it out, Senator, that's twelve grand a year. Maybe that's small change to you but not to our family," Barbara said. "My husband and I are fully employed. We have a four-year-old child and just get by on two salaries. We already pay huge insurance premiums, but what is covered falls far short of actual drug costs."

"I understand your frustration, Ms. Simon, but drug manufacturers have costs too, you know," Shank said.

"Look Senator, insulin has been manufactured for a very long time. It's not a new, fancy drug," Simon said. "I'm not an economist but I can figure out production costs couldn't have gone up that much. According to the American Diabetes Association, there are over seven million people in this country who need insulin for their diabetes. That's a big market for one drug. They don't *need* to raise prices. They do it because they know they can get away with it."

Shank knew he'd met his match. Further questions would expose him as an unfeeling misanthrope, something most politicians, with some notable exceptions, try to avoid.

"Thank you, Ms. Simon for coming. We'll take what you said into consideration as we study this new legislation," Shank said.

***

More than three hundred fifty miles northeast of Washington DC, in Middlesex County Massachusetts Courthouse, the Attorney General's office concluded prosecution of Pylea Pharmaceutical's Chief Executive Officer, one Reginald Warner, his Board of Directors and several other high-placed Pylea executives, giving the pharmaceutical industry more bad press.

At WKVC-TV, "New England's Choice for News," their news analysis team was dissecting the attorney general's suit against Pylea. The jury had found every single defendant guilty on all counts.

"Letitia, can you take us through this tangled web so listeners can sort out the facts" Chet Durkin asked.

Letitia Jefferson, a graduate of Harvard Law School, was a Black no-nonsense legal reporter. She'd written for local newspapers and was a fixture at WKVC for over fifteen years. Her round face, tightly woven hair, and contralto voice were familiar to New England audiences. Like others on this award-winning team, she was widely admired for her candor, intelligence and incisiveness.

"The issues boiled down to price gouging, price fixing, bribery, and advocating for non-FDA-approved uses for Cidal, their blockbuster antibiotic," Letitia said. "They negotiated with Hempstead Institute, which holds the patent for Cidal, to produce and market it. But Pylea was free to set the price, with Hempstead getting a percentage of the profits. Hempstead, importantly, is held blameless for all that went on in this suit."

"What is Cidal and what price had Pylea set for it?"

"Cidal is a new antibiotic that knocks out resistant bacterial organisms that cause hospital-acquired infections, often after surgery. Pylea priced the so-called kit -- antibiotic and paraphernalia needed to administer it -- at $500,000 per treatment."

"A half-million dollars per treatment? Did I hear you right?"

"You did. The defense arguments are typical in cases like this. They claim expenses involved in research, development and marketing justify this cost. They contend drug companies have success with some drugs and some failures, so when they have a successful drug, profits from it offset losses for others. They say this is how drug manufacturers can continue to discover life-saving drugs for the world."

"David Frer, you teach at the business school. What do you think of those arguments?"

"That theory is business 101. But-- and this is a big 'but'-- that price is a real outlier. Drugs this expensive are usually those known as "orphan" drugs, meaning they are for rare diseases. They do cost a lot to develop and there is a tiny market for them, so the profit in making them is small. I know of no other antibiotic that comes close to $500,000 per treatment. And Pylea had nothing to do with its development. That took place at the Hempstead Institute. I agree with the jury verdict that this was price gouging."

"Then there was the issue of price-fixing," Chet said. "Jorge Rodriquez, please chime in with your thoughts."

"The evidence presented by the attorney general's lawyer was damning. Subpoenaed emails and phone records between Warner and insurance executives from Old Forge and Winger couldn't have been more convincing," Rodriquez said. "They openly discussed transferring stocks to family members, stating their companies couldn't receive stock directly because such transactions would be seen on their books. Acknowledging that clearly made them culpable when they committed their companies to paying the exorbitant amount Warner set in exchange for stocks."

"We have to take a break," Chet announced. "Our call-in number is on the screen. We'd love to hear from you, our viewers. We'll be back with more."

The panel members chatted among themselves while commercials -- ironically, many for drugs -- danced on the studio monitors. Chet told Letitia that when the program resumed, he wanted her to dive right into the physician bribery issue.

"There were two more issues the lawsuit named," Letitia began. "The first was bribery of a couple of infectious disease specialists from two famous academic hospitals. These doctors were prominent nationally and internationally, known for their publications and for frequent lectures to physicians at conferences worldwide."

"You mention bribery. How were they bribed? That's serious," David Frer said.

"They were given, among other things, long family vacations in Hawaii for promoting Cidal as a panacea for hospital acquired resistant bugs. They heralded its introduction with such phrases as 'can't wait until it's available' or 'it can't get into our hands fast enough.' Not exactly the kind of scientific objectivity one hopes for."

Chet turned to Jorge Rodriquez. "The jury found them guilty of something else, right Jorge?"

"Well, this last thing was a little more borderline, but the jury was on a roll. The sales reps for Pylea were already touting Cidal not only for proven resistant organisms, but as a routine antibiotic for all infections seen in the hospital and even as a drug to be used prophylactically in surgical cases. These were not FDA approved uses for this drug. I spoke with a couple of infectious disease specialists who told me that if you want to destroy an antibiotic's effectiveness, overuse is a sure way to do that. So that's not a good long-range strategy. Apparently, the leaders at Pylea were interested only in short-term profit. By the time resistance to this antibiotic would have emerged, the Pylea high command would have been retired billionaires."

The call-in coordinator at WKVC-TV placed a heap of messages in front of Chet. When Jorge finished his sentence, Chet picked up the first note.

"This is from one of our viewers. 'Have the drug-makers gone mad? If people can't afford their drugs and they stop buying them, they won't make *any* money. Talk about killing the goose that lays golden eggs." And here's another: "I work for a drug company and have to say these are exceptions. Most of us in this business really work hard to bring safe and effective drugs to people needing them." And this: "I'm glad these pirates are getting their just deserts. I hope they get long prison terms, so they have lots of time to contemplate their sins."

"Now I'd like to welcome Kathy McClelland to the discussion. Kathy, you followed the criminal case against Reginald Warner. Fill us in on those trials."

"Mr. Warner will be sentenced next month. As you know, he killed a man's dog while trespassing on a property. He was convicted for destruction of personal property, not a felony, but he lost also on the voyeurism trial brought by Dina Robbins," McClelland said. "The police also won on resisting arrest charges and leaving the scene of a crime. He's facing jail time for several things. How long is up in the air. Of course, his lawyers are appealing all the guilty verdicts. This could drag on for some time."

"Is he out on bail?"

"Yes, over a million dollars bail. Flight is not considered likely with bail that high. His comments to the press after both trials were that he'd be exonerated on appeal. He seemed confident that would happen."

"Sorry, our time is short. There are hearings in congress going on right now on pharmaceutical practices. We'll bring those stories to you when they break. Until next time, stay tuned for all the news on WKVC, New England's Choice for News."

Chapter 38

Tom was preoccupied with the high drama of hearings in Washington and Warner's riveting trials in Boston, so Gwen Allen's opioid addiction problem drifted into a background haze. He woke after a night of restless sleep, a kaleidoscope of memories whirling in his mind, reminding him of those endless weeks after his return from the Middle East War when invasive dreams were nightly occurrences. He reasoned those recent events, piled on top of one another, had exceeded a saturation set point and overflowed. Once awake, Gwen popped up to first place on his list of things to worry about.

When she answered his phone call, he was relieved to find she'd been "clean" for a month in an effective rehab program. She was pleased too, and proud she'd won her addiction battle.

"I feel like I've pulled myself out of a deep rabbit hole where everything seemed like an Alice experience. Been watching the news about Purdue and Insys and realize that I'm only one of millions snagged in this net. I feel so lucky I haven't become one of those statistics, you know, dead from accidental overdose or suicide."

"Obviously, I couldn't be happier for you," Tom said. "Congratulations on your accomplishment. You're lucky, but more than that, you were determined.

"The reason I called is that I heard about a consolidation of opioid cases in an Ohio court. Most plaintiffs are local governments trying to get reimbursement for money spent for addiction services provided in their communities. As I understand it, there are also some individuals joining the suits," Tom said. "As I find out more, I'll let you know how to add your name as a plaintiff. The other thing we'll watch for, and you should keep your eyes open for this as well, are class action suits against manufacturers of opioids. You should join these if they come about."

"I met a public interest lawyer at the rehab center," Gwen said. "She's been working on cases pro bono for a couple of years. She knows a lot about what's happening. I'll tell her about the Ohio thing, but I bet she's aware of it. Please let me know if you hear anything new. I'd like some recompense for my suffering, but more importantly, I'm committed to making sure this doesn't happen to others.

"Thanks for calling, Tom."

***

As daylight crept into his condo and his call to Gwen swept away the cobwebs of his dreams, Tom's heart slowed. After tossing down some yogurt and decaf coffee he tapped into his favorite music station streaming on his computer. Despite impatience for music to resume after several commercials, one ad grabbed his attention.

"If you want robotic surgery, why not come to the world's best robotic surgery center? Go to our website for more information at EasternRegionRobotics.com today."

Robotic surgery? I've heard of it but thought it was a passing fad. I doubt many surgeons would get involved in it. But... could a one-armed surgeon learn how to do it? He went to their website. What he saw opened his eyes wide. Photographs from actual robots performing surgical procedures on live human beings. *This is for real.* Then he saw a tab: "For Fellowships in Robotic Surgery, call the number on your screen."

Why not? What do I have to lose?

He called and followed the inevitable telephone tree. He pressed "5" when prompted leading to a message about fellowships in robotic surgery and still another telephone number listed for "further information." Frustrating, but he pushed the flash key and dialed the number.

"Eastern Region Robotics. This is Celia, how may I help you?"

"This is Dr. Tom Barrett. I'm a Board-Certified surgeon and I'm interested in information on training in robotic surgery. Can you help me?"

"Yes sir, I can help you. Give me your name and contact information. I'll send you information and appropriate applications for the fellowship."

"That would be great. Can you tell me a little bit about it? For example, what qualifications does one need to apply? How long is it? Cost? Things like that."

"You said you're Board Certified in surgery and that's requirement number one. The fellowship lasts two years and we pay a small stipend. All applicants are required to have a personal interview with Dr. Johannsen, our fellowship director. The next available fellowship starts July first."

"Sounds interesting. Please send the application forms to me," he said, giving her his email address.

The prospect of getting back into an operating room, breathing in its antiseptic smell, was like having a curtain drawn aside allowing a view of a brightly lit path forward. Tom let out several hoots of exhilaration. *Good thing I'm home and not in the office where people would think I'd lost my mind. Maybe I have. How would the one-armed thing work? Would I have to give up PharmaTruth? Who'd replace me there?* He paced around his condo, eager to explore this newly discovered opportunity. He scanned his browser for more information and spent most of his day researching robotic surgery.

***

The application popped up on his email towards the end of the day. Tom would have to dig out documents he'd long since buried in boxes, but he was pumped and eager to complete the forms and send them off. He was even more anxious to tell Cynthia.

Since Nassau, Cynthia had moved many of her things to his condo, but she kept her place in Worcester for those long days at the nursing school. She had barely gotten through the door that evening when Tom threw his arm around her and gave her a long, lingering kiss. When he relaxed his hold, she backed away slightly, looking at him quizzically.

"Okay, what's up? I love it when you greet me like that, but it doesn't happen every night, so you have something to tell me. Good news, right?"

"No, just news. It could be good, but I won't know for a while." He told her about the fellowship.

"That is big news alright. Wow. I have a lot of questions, but I doubt you have answers yet. How does robotic surgery work? And how would you participate in it?"

"The business end of the robot is in the operating room positioned over the patient. The surgeon sits at a console in the operating room, or even in another room, with a computer, a camera and controls that operate the robotic arms as they do the actual operating," Tom said, getting more enthusiastic as he spoke.

"Say this is a thoracic procedure. A 3D camera is inserted into the patient's chest cavity through a small incision showing the inside of the chest cavity. Robotic instruments that are engineered to move in all directions are inserted through other tiny incisions. These instruments are controlled by the surgeon sitting at the console. Diseased tissue or tissue for biopsy can be removed by the robotic arm. This same approach can be used for many other areas of the body. It's sort of an extension of the concept of laparoscopic surgery."

"So, the surgeon is still performing the surgery, only remotely?"

"Yeah, but from what I've read, the surgeon at the console can see the surgical field much better with the camera than through our surgical incision. My right hand still will be the operating hand at the console. Either another surgeon or some other arrangement, such as a pedal that I would control with my foot, can run the left-hand robotic arm."

"Sounds so exciting. What's your next step?"

"Well, the first hurdle is filling out a mountain of application papers. Then, supposing I get this fellowship, which is a big 'if' right now, it lasts two years. I didn't ask the biggest question -- my arm. I'm sure the woman I talked to couldn't have answered it. I'll ask when I get an interview. But the big dilemma is that I'd have to give up what I'm doing at PharmaTruth. I love that work, but I miss surgery so much."

"I think it's a great idea. You've been married to surgery as long as I've known you. It's your primal love. But, you know, a lot of people are depending on what PharmaTruth is trying to do. What are your thoughts about preserving all the work you've done there? And having it continue?"

She looked at Tom and could tell by the sparkle in his eyes and his general animation how important this new opportunity to wade into uncharted territory was to him. Cynthia's eyes dampened as she gazed, seeing the Tom Barrett she knew when he was a fresh-faced surgical intern, and she was head nurse at Boston Medical Center Emergency Room.

"Why don't you try to talk to the director before you fill out application forms to see if your" -- she stumbled over the words -- "your disability would disqualify you for robotic surgery. I don't know much about it, but it seems to me it might require both hands."

"I worried about that too, but I'm hoping that manufacturers of robots might be able to adapt the equipment for me to use it. This will be the first thing I ask when I interview."

"It's so good seeing you excited again. But I know how committed you are to PharmaTruth too. I guess we can procrastinate about its future until you know what's possible in this fellowship."

"Yes, I am committed to PharmaTruth, but you know, I don't have to oversee it. I mean, others would be better administrators than I've been and besides, even though I like blazing new trails, once the trail is laid out, others can walk it. I'm content to watch it grow and do its good works without being its commander in chief. Just being the founder is satisfying."

They looked at each other, neither wanting to venture further into this unknown terrain. Cynthia worried that Tom's hopes might be dashed if he were rejected because of his paralysis. But she also knew that the world was changing and people with various limitations were finding new acceptance in all walks of life. Adaptations of tools, machinery, and automobiles were in wide use so why not use the knowledge and skills of a highly trained and competent surgeon?

"This is Dr. Barrett calling again," Tom said, the following morning. "Thanks for sending that application. I need to find a lot of supporting documents," he said, putting off the real reason for his call. "Is there a deadline for getting this to you?"

"The cutoff date is two months from now," Celia said.

"One further question," Tom said. "Would it be possible to talk to the director, either by phone or in person before I complete my application? I have a specific reason for needing to do this." He hoped she wouldn't ask what that was.

"I'll ask Dr. Johanssen to call you. He's tied up in surgery this morning but has time to call after lunch. I'll give him your message."

"Thank you," Tom said. *What does the world of surgeons think about this innovation? Are they threatened by it? Is robotic surgery considered to be a gimmick, something that will flare and then sputter? Or is it the wave of the future?*

He told Dolores he'd be working at home for the next few days and to call with major issues. He browsed around the internet and studied everything he could find about robotic surgery. He called several erstwhile surgical colleagues and got varying opinions, most of them positive.

"Dr. Barrett, this is Dr. Johanssen calling. My secretary told me you're interested in our fellowship, and you have a specific question for me. I'd be happy to try to answer it."

Tom was impressed with his warm manner and identified his accent as distinctively Minnesotan.

"Yes, I was trained in trauma surgery at Boston Medical several years ago. I'm in my late thirties and have not operated for about five years due to an injury that paralyzed my left arm. Before I apply for your fellowship, I need to know whether that would disqualify me." Tom exhaled, having gotten his statement out. He waited for what he considered a long time for Johanssen's answer.

"You should come to see me, and we'll talk. Yours is an unusual request, first time it's come up, so I need to discuss this with you in person." He paused, warming to the challenge. "A very interesting situation, one with distinct possibilities. Make an appointment."

Tom arranged a time to see Johanssen, his mind still racing, He then turned back to his research. After two ten-hour days of that, he was satisfied that robotic surgery was legitimate avant-garde medicine. It was broadening its scope of applications each year. It made him even more desirous to get into action.

Chapter 39

Senator Blake banged down his cherry gavel, calling the senate finance committee to order, continuing hearings on the Brill-Rafferty Affordable Drugs Act.

"Although our first group of witnesses were called 'consumers,' today we have a doctor who, although not a consumer himself, will tell us about things that are happening behind the scenes that ultimately affect consumers. Practicing physicians write prescriptions for drugs we're discussing so it's appropriate to hear from one. Dr. Norman Wise, please take the witness chair."

Norman Wise carried his notes, sat down and adjusted a small microphone mounted in front of him. He stated his name in his deep baritone and read a prepared statement.

"Senators, as a doctor taking an oath to do no harm, I'm ashamed of actions I'm about to describe. I hope my telling you these things will make you aware of what happens in some parts of the drug industry and why new legislation is needed to stop these abuses. In addition, I hope my testimony serves as a cautionary tale to my fellow physicians who could slide down this slippery slope.

"I became acquainted with a detail man, what drug salespersons are often called, who came regularly to my cardiology practice in Boston to promote heart medications his company made. He was an affable man -- let's call him Jim -- and I welcomed seeing him. He was generous with samples of his company's heart drugs that I passed on to patients on limited incomes, thinking I could help them this way. Because of my perceived friendship with Jim, I naturally prescribed the drugs he provided to me as samples."

Wise cleared his throat, drank a few sips of water and resumed. He described his lectures and the bogus research studies he participated in, as well as his activity of prescribing off-label uses of some drugs and prescribing opioids to more and more patients.

"There followed an attrition of my rational thinking, a progression to becoming a so-called 'targeted doctor,' one who could easily be influenced. Drug salespeople manipulated me and other malleable doctors into prescribing opioids to patients in ever increasing amounts. It rose to a point where I was prescribing more opioids in a week than most mainstream doctors would prescribe in a year." Wise's face sagged the longer he spoke. "The number of patients in my practice who begged me for additional opioid prescriptions skyrocketed. Then the nightmare came: drug overdoses and suicides among my patients. I realized I couldn't go on or I would end up on an autopsy table myself."

Wise continued, glancing up at the row of stern-faced senators sitting behind their nameplates. He reached for more water and wiped some sweat from his forehead. Committee members were sharply attentive now, realizing the doctor had crossed a bright line in his relationship with the drug company.

"That's why I'm here," Wise said in a mournful voice. "I'll undoubtedly lose my license because of this testimony.

I'll probably be sued. But I can't live with the guilt any longer."

He stopped. His head hung down, his shoulders slumped, and tears streaked his face.

The hearing room was as quiet as a catacomb. World-weary senators whose tenure was long and who thought they'd heard it all were chilled with a spectral vision of doctors paid to addict patients to medicines ostensibly designed and manufactured to relieve pain. Cameras had stopped taking pictures. The media stopped taking notes. Minutes passed before Senator Blake pulled his microphone toward his face.

"Dr. Wise, on behalf of the committee, I thank you for coming here. I know this has been painful for you. I respect you for telling us your story."

Blake allowed minutes to tick by to let the full impact of Wise's confessions be absorbed.

"Does anyone on the committee wish to ask Dr. Wise a question?"

"Doctor Wise, I have a question," Senator DeVore said, leaning forward over his microphone. "Didn't you ever question what was going on? Didn't you realize what was happening, that you were being used? It seems you should have been aware sooner that you were sinking into unprofessional and duplicitous activity."

"Senator, you're right. I should have seen what was happening, and at some level I did feel soiled. But by then I was deep into this, and I rationalized. It's analogous to the story about frogs used in scientific experiments," Wise said. "Perhaps you remember this analogy of tossing a frog into boiling water. It will make enormous effort to jump right out. But if you put him into cool water and gradually turn the heat up, the frog will accommodate to this gentle rise in temperature, until the high temperature kills the frog. That's what it was like for me."

Senator Blake looked to his right and to his left, saw no other hands raised.

"Committee hearing is adjourned until two o'clock."

***

Cynthia skirted around a gaggle of reporters outside the hearing chamber, worried one of them might discover she was to testify next and pummel her with questions. She was escorted to her seat just before Senator Blake tapped his gavel for resumption. Blake asked her to identify herself, swore her in, and then asked her to tell the committee why she was there.

"My name is Cynthia Billings. I spent eight years as head nurse in the emergency department at Boston Medical Center and am currently dean of the school of nursing at Commonwealth University in Worcester Massachusetts," Cynthia then said in a steady voice. "In my hospital work I contracted hepatitis C from numerous hypodermic needle sticks, a common occupational hazard for health care workers." She stopped for some water. Her mouth was dry, and she was surprised how anxious she felt.

"Please continue with your story, Ms. Billings," Senator Blake said.

"Thank you, Senator.

"For two years I had frequent bouts of fatigue and mild jaundice, yellowing of the skin. My blood test for hepatitis C antibody came back positive and my liver function studies were abnormal. My doctor advised me to get the highly effective medications for hepatitis C."

Senator DeVore raised his hand and Blake asked Cynthia to interrupt her testimony for a question.

"How effective is medication in treating hepatitis?" DeVore asked.

"It has a nincty-percent cure rate," she said, confidence rising as she testified.

"That's phenomenal. Was a United States drug company involved in the development of these drugs?"

"Yes."

"That demonstrates what our terrific American drug industry has been doing for years. They've given us so many drugs to treat, and in many cases, wipe out diseases," DeVore said. "Only in a free society such as ours could this have been accomplished."

"I agree, Senator, with your statement about the many accomplishments of pharmaceutical companies. We are a healthier population because of their efforts. But there's more to it than that," she said. "The drug for treating hepatitis C was found by a scientist who had previously worked with the Department of Veterans' Affairs, a federally funded agency. His small company developed the drug and sold the patent and the monopoly rights to the company now charging this high price."

"We can all agree that we're blessed with new medicines developed by pharmaceutical companies, both here and in other countries around the world," Senator Blake said. "But your story, Ms. Billings, illustrates that, like most things in our world, the full story is often more complicated than it appears."

With that polite dismissal of DeVore's overzealous patriotism, he turned back to Cynthia.

"Ms. Billings, tell us what happened next."

"Well, I was surprised by what happened next. I have excellent health insurance through my job at the nursing school, but I heard drug treatment for hepatitis C wasn't always fully covered, so I checked with the insurance company. I was turned down. Why? I had no proof of liver fibrosis either by biopsy or liver elastography, another test of liver damage. In other words, my liver had to show extensive damage, or my policy wouldn't cover treatment."

Senator DeVore interrupted again.

"Ms. Billings, if you don't have serious liver damage it seems to me the insurance company is perfectly justified in not covering treatment. Sounds like your disease is pretty mild."

"Senator, my disease is a ticking time bomb. It could get worse tomorrow. This is anxiety-producing, to say the least. And the cost of my treatment for severe liver failure would far outpace the cost of early prevention."

Cynthia paused and looked up at this array of senators before her and focused on DeVore. *Was his low level of understanding and sympathy representative of the others on this committee? Did these senators know anything about hepatitis C?* She decided to slip into her teaching mode.

"Senators, hepatitis C is a major public health problem. Three and a half million people in the United States have these viruses in their blood. Half don't know they're diseased because they have no symptoms. Some will go on to cirrhosis requiring expensive long-term care, a huge burden on our health care system."

"But do we know that all will go on to cirrhosis?" Senator DeVore pressed.

"No, we can't know that," Cynthia conceded. "But when you have a drug that can prevent that progression in at least some patients, how many of you would choose to be the doctor or nurse telling a patient that they have a disease for which there's a treatment that is 90% effective, but the catch is that they have to come up with about $84,000 for full treatment if their insurance won't cover it?"

It did seem like a couple of committee members squirmed when she mentioned the price tag.

"But isn't it true that the pharmaceutical industry has gone the extra mile to ease this problem by creating various drug assistance programs available to patients?" De Vore said. "I've been informed there are ways around having to pay that much. In fact, most patients don't have to pay anywhere near that because of coupons and rebates and other assistance programs."

"Let me tell you a little bit about that," Cynthia said. "With some drugs, not necessarily for hepatitis C but for a lot of others, when an assistance program kicks in, some patients pay nothing. You're right about that. The reason? The cost for some drugs is transferred to Medicare. Medicare can't negotiate prices so that program ends up paying the sticker price, the whole price set by the drug manufacturers. The result is a steadily and rapidly rising health care budget paid for by -- guess who. Taxpayers. And what do you think will happen with that? Some politicians will argue that Medicare is going to go bust and we need to restrict it or get rid of it. Partly because Medicare can't negotiate drug prices.

"In the case of hepatitis C drugs, private insurers have developed aggressive prior authorization systems to avoid coverage of this expensive treatment, the price of which is set by drug companies. Even Medicare and Medicaid are becoming more restrictive. Patients incur costs, co-pays or co-insurance, determined by pharmacy plans."

"But isn't a crucial role being played by program benefits managers?" DeVore insisted. "They negotiate millions of dollars of savings for their clients, right?"

"Program benefits managers do play a central role in this, but not what your question implies. Nearly all drugs they manage are cheaper generics, so it has nothing to do with hepatitis C treatment, which has no generic alternative. But since you brought it up, Senator, I must tell you that some program benefits managers are a problem in the larger arena of drug pricing. They act as middlemen and skim off the difference between a lower price they set for pharmacies and their much larger charge to Medicaid. Taxpayers are again the losers here." *Does anyone here care about that corruption? I hope my testifying helps move the needle towards not putting up with this, but the committee looks half-asleep. Except for this blowhard.*

"What about all those coupon deals?" DeVore persisted, now shrill, with color flooding his cheeks.

"Manufacturer's coupons are always for high priced brand name drugs and are time-limited. When the time limit runs out, the patient, afraid to change from a familiar drug to one she knows little about, will continue to buy the drug she's used to, now without a coupon discount."

"Ms. Billings, let's return to the issue about hepatitis C treatment," Senator Blake interjected. "We've strayed a little from that, although we appreciate hearing what you've said about program benefits managers, a topic we should take up later."

"Thank you, Senator Blake. I've talked about insurance coverage for hepatitis C drugs. Take Medicaid as an example of a government-sponsored program. There are so many different coverage options in Medicaid that availability of treatment and what it costs boils down to which state you live in," she said. "And that's being further threatened by some politicians who want to return Medicaid to a block grant program.

"There's no question that the patchwork quilt of coverage for hepatitis C drugs is a problem, but the root problem -- I can't emphasize this enough -- is the high price set by manufacturers.

"Right now, given today's price for hepatitis C drugs, if we chose to treat all 3.5 million chronically infected people in the United States it would cost 310 billion dollars. I'll say that again: 310 billion dollars. That price tag would ultimately be met by rapidly rising insurance premiums paid by ordinary people."

Several of the senators looked up when they heard this. One thing that always gets elected legislators' attention, Cynthia knew, is explaining outlays of large sums of money to voters.

"What is desperately needed is very simple: substantial lowering of drug prices and uniform payment by all third parties.

"Thank you for listening." Cynthia folded her notes, took a drink of water, and waited for questions. She didn't have to wait long.

"What about uninsured people who have little money?" Senator Blake asked.

"Uninsured individuals must make less than about $50,000 annually to get financial assistance. For a family of two, less than about $68,000. In our economy, that's considered borderline income.

"Thank you, Ms. Billings," Blake said. "Other questions?" Committee members sat stone-faced. Cynthia couldn't read their thoughts. She was sure of one thing: DeVore hated her for speaking truth to power, but she took great satisfaction that her answers were based on facts instead of slogans.

"There being no more questions, I want to thank Ms. Billings for educating us on these issues. It will help as we move forward in our deliberations."

Cynthia plied her way through the crowd, waving off microphones and chattering reporters, and headed toward where she was to meet Tom.

"Great job, Cyn. I'm so proud of you." He gave her a hug and whisked her away to a waiting driver.

Chapter 40

Eastern Region Robotics was affiliated with a major academic medical center in bustling downtown Boston.

After being away from hospitals for some years, Tom was awed by the enormity of this complex. Its hyperactivity was fueled by the quickness of step of men and women in scrubs, long white lab coats, stethoscopes wound around their shoulders, and synthetic blue bags tied over their shoes. The lines at registration desks were populated by every size, shape, color, and age of patients, with words of many languages filling the air. Tom breathed in mixed aromas of coffee, food, garlic, and body odor. He'd forgotten the milieu of large hospital reception areas.

Once he got off the elevator, he walked for what seemed like a city block before finding Eastern Robotics. On its futuristic glass door was engraved a list of donors, who must have been quite generous, judging by the upscale décor. He introduced himself to a receptionist and was welcomed warmly. She offered him coffee and led him into Dr. Johanssen's office.

Tom wiped his moist right hand on his trousers. Then Tom's leg started involuntary jiggling, an old tic he thought no longer part of his repertoire of nerves. *Why am I so anxious? This is like those interviews for residency ten years ago. I should've outgrown this kind of angst.* As he ruminated about this, Dr. Johanssen stepped quietly into the room.

"You must be Tom Barrett," he said, looking straight into Tom's eyes. "I'm Oliver Johanssen. Very nice to meet you."

"R-right," Tom stammered. "Good to meet you as well."

"So, I read over your CV. Very impressive. But tell me about yourself. I'm intrigued by your arm issue and what robotic surgery might offer you."

"How much time do you have?" Tom laughed.

"As much as we need. I have no patients this afternoon."

Tom told him about his service in the Middle East, his PTSD, his experiences at Zylinski, his head injury that led to his arm paralysis, the legal settlement, and his current work with PharmaTruth.

"But what I miss most is operating. It was only when I saw your website that I realized how much I missed it. I'm questioning whether robotics might fill this void."

"Well, I've made some inquiries since I talked with you and I have some good news, I think. Ian McGregor, one of our engineers, got excited when I told him about your situation and came up with a plan -- a possible application," Johanssen said. "Your right arm is still your dominant arm, right?"

"Yes, I've always been right-handed."

"He said he thought he could 'rig up' -- his words for a complex piece of engineering -- a model that would employ your right arm as the 'operating' arm, and the left arm run either by a human assistant or some other arrangement. This obviously would take time to implement but he thought it was eminently possible. He'd like to work with you to bring this about."

Tom's heart was racing, and he was fighting back tears. Like the movie line, "There's no crying in baseball," he didn't think tearing up would be received well. When he was sure his voice wouldn't quiver, he said, "I couldn't be happier," and then blurted, "When can we start?"

"I think soon, but I'll have to talk more to Ian. It will probably involve your working with him and other designers at the factory to develop a satisfactory model. I don't know how long that would take."

"Where's their factory? Would I have to move?"

"Maynard. Where do you live?"

"Beacon Hill. Maynard's great, within easy commuting distance. I was worried it was in California or someplace distant."

"Let me talk to Ian and I'll call you."

"Does this mean I have a fellowship?"

"Oh, yes, sorry. I thought that was evident. Of course, you need to fill out the paperwork. It's a special fellowship, earmarked for a doctor with a disability, supported by an anonymous donor. I know you don't need money, but this donor insisted. If you want to pass it on to your non-profit, that's okay with her."

"I can't thank you enough, Dr. Johanssen. And the donor, whoever she is. This is so, I don't know, exhilarating."

"You know, Tom, robotics is in its infancy. It's your unique situation that opens new pathways. Thank you for giving us this chance to expand."

Tom hurried out of the building to call Cynthia. This was a cause to celebrate, a rebirth, a time for toasts and high fives.

Chapter 41

A buzz filled the corridor outside the committee hearing chamber. This was the day pharmaceutical executives were scheduled. News media smelled blood in the water. Headlines had trumpeted the compelling testimony of consumer witnesses. Their stories were pure human interest, with testimony by Cynthia Billings that was evidence-based as well as personal.

The CEO's arrived together in a Mercedes van, not good public relations, their arrogance smothering good sense. Four white middle-aged men in almost identical dark blue suits, pale blue shirts and tightly knotted small-patterned ties, marched single file into the chamber. They sat in a row, their tables equipped with tiny microphones on flexible necks. Seeming to move as one, they said nothing to each other, looked neither right nor left, like bloodless automatons.

Senator Blake was already seated when Senators Martz and DeVore entered and stopped to whisper into Blake's ear. He nodded and turned back to his notes. Martz looked pale and thin. Rumors had it that he was dying of cancer, but he hadn't acknowledged any illness. DeVore also looked pale, but his pallor was his normal complexion that complemented his thin frame, gray eyes and permanent frown. His fingers were long and spidery as they moved noiselessly over his notes.

Senator Blake called the session to order, then called Herbert Daly, CEO from Dartos Pharmaceuticals. After he was sworn in, he read from his prepared statement.

"Thank you, Senators, for an opportunity to comment on this impending legislation. I've been asked by my colleagues," he stretched his arm to indicate three other men seated next to him, "to read our combined statement. We'll all be available for questions."

Blake looked at the committee members to get their approval on this proposal. Seeing no dissent, he nodded to Daly.

"I'll start with the first paragraph, which advocates requiring drug manufacturers to negotiate their prices with federal agencies. May I remind the committee that current statutes prevent such negotiations. We support preservation of those statutes. The drug industry makes every effort to set fair prices and new laws requiring negotiation of those prices would, in our view, be in violation of the American principle of minimal governmental control over commerce."

"Mr. Daly," Senator St. Clair interrupted, "are you aware that we need only to repeal existing legislation that bars Medicare from negotiating with the drug industry?"

"I defer to you to investigate that. But in my opinion that would be bad precedent," Daly replied.

"Well, it doesn't surprise me you think it would be bad precedent," St. Clair replied. "But most rational people agree we need both to lower drug prices and maintain Medicare for millions of people who depend on it for care and medications. Seems to me allowing price negotiations by Medicare would be bad precedent only for the drug makers."

"It would be bad for business across the board," Daly replied, with an edge. "Having increased government interference in business would be bad for the economy, bad for consumers, and bad for business."

"How so?" St. Clair persisted.

"It conflicts with our national principle of open competition," he shot back.

"Pardon me?" St. Clair jumped back in. "A bedrock principle of capitalism is that when more than one company makes a product, they compete to sell that product. One of the ways they compete is through pricing of their product. That kind of competition is supposed to make prices as low as possible. This principle's purpose, which your industry has repeatedly embraced in theory, is to set prices that are competitive and fair."

St. Clair paused and looked at Daly and his colleagues. He pulled his microphone closer so there would be no mistaking his next comment.

"You fellas are always carping about competition," St. Clair continued. "We need competition in setting prices for drugs in federal programs," he stated emphatically. "When everyone in the industry agrees on one price that thwarts fair pricing, competition doesn't really exist. Isn't that so?"

Daly was quiet. No reply he could conjure up wouldn't be argumentative, so he paused, looked down the line at his colleagues, whose faces were flushed, jaws set.

"Senator, are you implying that we're engaged in price-fixing?" he barked.

St. Clair paused to allow the question to be registered by all in the room. Then he said, in even tones, "There have been successful lawsuits against pharmaceutical companies, won because those companies had colluded to set prices for similar drugs at a similar level, Mr. Daly. You know that, the committee knows that, and citizens listening out there know that, so let's move on to the next item." St. Clair said with no mistaking his irritation.

Daly looked at his colleagues who had their eyes on their desks. He decided to cut his losses and move on to what he hoped was a stronger argument.

"The next paragraph discusses regulations capping out-of-pocket spending for drugs. Regulations like this involve serious government interference in free enterprise. This borders on socialism.

"The third paragraph of the proposed law introduces another extremely dangerous concept, that of importation of drugs from other countries. Manufacturing of drugs is a precise science and must be carefully done. Other countries don't have the regulations we have from the Food and Drug Administration. We must protect the American people against imported drugs that could be tainted, poorly compounded, or have incorrect dosages. The pharmaceutical industry emphatically opposes importation."

"Do you deny that around 40% of drugs available to patients in the United States are already made in some other country?" St. Clair asked.

"No, I don't deny that. But their importation is regulated by our FDA rules."

"So, you believe in regulation after all," exclaimed Senator St. Clair with a heavy dose of sarcasm. "That's good to hear. It seems to me that the same FDA that you endorse that regulates our US drug industry could just as well regulate drugs coming in from other countries."

"That's really complicated and would require a separate hearing to fully discuss," Daly said, shaking his head.

"I think the lawmakers on this committee, and in Congress in general, know a complicated issue when they see one," St. Clair fumed. "Of course, it would require study and that's exactly what this committee is here to do."

Daly struggled on in his tense testimony. He objected to the proposal about shortening time that patents would shield drug companies from competition by generic manufacturers, renewal of patents only when major changes were made to the drugs, restriction of direct advertising to consumers, and criminalizing hiring of doctors to advocate for particular drugs. His arguments were standard dogma and members of the committee had heard them all before.

St. Clair had his hand up again. Blake recognized him and Daly frowned as he anticipated more tough questions.

"I want to ask you about the so-called "nurse ambassadors" that some drug companies use. There was a lawsuit out west related to nurse ambassadors interfering with communication between doctors and patients to keep patients on particular drugs. Have you heard these complaints?"

"Yes, Senator, I've heard them."

"Well, what's the response of the drug industry?"

"There may have been a few rare instances where nurse ambassadors overstepped their responsibilities, but these professionally trained people have done great service for patients. I think it's a shame their mission has been smeared. Improving patients' lives is their passion."

"These stories keep coming out, Mr. Daly," St. Clair said, continuing to grill Daly. "They don't seem to be all that isolated. Perhaps attorneys general need to look into this. We've heard complaints from doctors about how these nurses appear to be accountable only to the drug companies, not to doctors who care for patients. We've been told that some of these nurses are getting kickbacks from drug companies to keep pushing drugs to patients."

"I can't comment on that, sir. Again, there may be isolated cases. Every business or profession has outliers who don't do what's right. But in the vast majority of cases nurse ambassadors make major contributions to patient care."

"Let me ask you about the drug industry's lobbying," changing the subject since he was getting no answers. "I'm told that between 1998 and 2004 there were nearly 1300 registered lobbyists who spent 900 million dollars to influence legislation dealing with the drug industry. The figure for 2018 alone is $281 million. The numbers of lobbyists must be higher than 1300 now, since that number is from two decades ago."

"I don't have current figures, but Senator, you know that there are lobbyists for every business, union, or profession, all advocating for the groups they work for to assure fair laws are passed that don't harm their industry. There's nothing wrong with that," Daly said.

"Nothing wrong unless it gives unfair advantage to an industry and penalizes people," St. Clair said. "The cost of lobbyists, all of whom are paid handsomely, is ultimately part of the cost of the product, in your case, drugs. I won't ask about your personal salary, but many drug executives make 20-30 million dollars each year. These salaries are borne by patients as well."

Daly squirmed in his chair, looked down the line to his cohorts, none looked back, looking straight ahead, probably glad they were not in Daly's seat, which was getting hotter the longer St. Clair questioned him.

"Let me ask you about political contributions. Millions of dollars are given to political candidates each year, three times as much going to one political party than to the other. What do you get for this investment?"

"Citizens of this country are allowed to contribute what they want to political parties. That's democracy in action."

"Industries aren't citizens, really, despite the Supreme Court's ludicrous decision. But that's another issue altogether," St. Clair growled. "And some would call this 'buying candidates' or more crudely, having them in their pockets, a sort of state capture."

Daly sat like a statue, any guilt about manipulating lawmakers didn't exist in his universe.

Senator St. Clair looked down at his notes for a moment, adjusting his glasses.

"Let's talk about advertising," he said, looking over his glasses. "On the rare occasions I watch television I can't get through an hour anymore without seeing several ads for drugs directed towards consumers. These ads don't really tell what the drugs do or what conditions they're supposed to treat. At the end of these ads an announcer spits out a litany of side effects in unintelligible rapid-fire language designed only to fulfill legal requirements and avoid liability, not to convey useful information.

"So, my question, Mr. Daly, is what percentage of the average drug manufacturer's budget goes into advertising and marketing? It must be expensive. TV ads are notoriously costly."

"Senator, it's so complicated and variable I can't possibly answer your question," Daly said, shaking his head. "I'm sorry."

"C'mon Mr. Daly, you're an executive of your company and you must have a handle on how your company spends its money. Your annual report to stockholders surely has a line item for that."

"As I said Senator, complicated and variable. I don't know the answer."

Senator Blake waited for Senator St. Clair to continue.

"I'm done with this witness," Senator St. Clair said as though he'd just inhaled a bad odor.

Blake looked at the other committee members and seeing no response from them, gaveled the session to a close. *What more could be said?* he thought.

Chapter 42

Reginald Warner was blazing mad. After his convictions, his handpicked Pylea board of directors unanimously fired him. Then they all abruptly resigned, desperate to escape being named in more suits. Pylea was put into court-ordered receivership and was up for sale. Warner's dreams of fabulous wealth had morphed into nightmares of sharing dank cells with foul-smelling, slack-jawed predatory men.

It's so unfair. I've done nothing wrong, other than being a visionary waving the flag for successful entrepreneurial spirit. The worst of it is all that money I've pissed away to lawyers to keep me out of jail. All appeals to Warner's convictions had been denied. He was due in court to face sentencing in a couple of weeks.

Pulling on a light jacket, Warner went to his condo safe and took out the million dollars he'd hidden before everything hit the fan. He was glad that long ago he'd put his ten million dollars severance pay from Drum Pharmaceuticals in a bank in Grand Cayman. Once he was out of the United States, he could draw that out. He'd sold his Ferrari after the dog incident and bought a non-descript car, already strategizing his escape if he lost his appeals. A sketchy character in Revere fabricated a fake passport for him since he'd forfeited his passport along with his bail money. His counterfeit passport name was Bill Reynolds.

Warner smiled with satisfaction at his plan to elude authorities. *That judge, who figured I wasn't a flight risk because of the high bail…what a stupid bastard.*

He would drive to Texas and cross the border into Mexico. Picking the best place to cross was key to a clean escape. He chose Rio Grande City, where an international bridge would take him to Camargo, Tamaulipas. Before anyone found out he'd skipped he'd be high in a mountain retreat he knew from his years of working in Texas. He would then depart quietly into South America and get lost.

Setting out from Cambridge early the next morning, Warner ditched his old electronic gear. He bought a new cellphone with a fictitious name through his Revere passport forger. He decided to follow the interstates south, forsaking blue highways, even though they might be less patrolled. Commuter traffic on an interstate offered more anonymity than back roads. *It will be easier to hide in a crowd. Might be dangerous to get pulled over by a hayseed cop in some Podunk town for a minor infraction.* He had his pistol if he needed to use it to avoid getting cornered.

For twelve hours Warner drove. He grabbed a hamburger and fries from a diner and continued for another four hours. A no-tell motel on the outskirts of a small town in North Carolina was the perfect resting point. Paying cash for a room, he told the sleepy clerk he'd be leaving early the next morning. Warner dropped into bed and went to sleep as though he were an innocent puppy. The sky was still a dusky gray when he awoke after four hours. Dressing quickly, he was on the road for another long day.

On the day of his exodus from life as he'd known it, the sun was bright, the sky a brilliant azure, blinding even with sunglasses. Warner fell in behind a long column of cars, trucks, buses and motorcycles on a ramp inching toward Camargo International Bridge. He chose rush hour so he'd be less conspicuous, hoping a crushing crowd would dull the senses of functionaries whose job was to inspect credentials and wave people through the tedious process of passing an arbitrary boundary between countries. As he crawled toward the booth where judgment would be rendered, he felt a twinge in his chest. Despite the air-conditioner on full blast he began to sweat profusely. *Get a grip. This'll be over in a few minutes, and I'll be free.*

"Passport please," a blue uniform said.

Warner handed him his fake passport with sweating hands.

"Gonna get any hotter?" Warner said, hoping to befriend someone who could change his life.

"Always does. What's the purpose of your trip?"

"Vacation," Warner said with conviction. "Been lookin' forward to this for six months."

"Mr. Reynolds, pull your car over to that parking space."

Panic caused a surge of acid to rise in his esophagus.

"What for, officer?"

"Need to look in your trunk and check out your car."

Warner considered questioning him further but thought better of it. *Do as they say, don't raise suspicion.*

Another officer came out of the booth and told Warner in cop-speak to "exit the vehicle." He got out, pulled a cigarette from his pocket and lit it with shaking hands. *What the hell is goin' on here? Is there method in their search?* He watched the cop open the trunk, lift out his bags and proceed to dig through them. He did the same with Warner's other bags, placing them on the ground behind the car. Another younger cop who looked like he was about 14, came out of the shed with a low cart on wheels. He sprawled his skinny body onto it and rolled under the car. Warner was getting faint in the heat and asked one of the guards if he could use the restroom in the guardhouse.

"Out of order in there. You'll have to hold it.

"Let me see your passport again."

"Sure." Warner handed it over.

The guard looked at Warner, then again at the passport, then once more at Warner. The kid emerged from under the car and came over to Warner.

"You got a bad muffler under there," he said. He turned and faced the other cop. "Nothing under there I could see."

"Officer, can I get back in the car? I'm not feeling well." His face was red from heat and sweat showed under his arms and down the middle of the back of his shirt.

The guard looked at him, flipped his sunglasses off, grabbed his arm and led him into the guardhouse.

"Lie down on this leather couch. I'll get you some water," he said.

Warner felt his heart thundering against his chest. He felt his head was about to explode. Lying down eased some of his chest pain, but he felt he was going to vomit. *Must be that lousy hamburger and fries from that damned diner last night.* One of the guards approached him holding a blood pressure cuff. He wrapped it around his arm and checked it.

"Your pressure is sky high," he said. "Are you on pills for high blood pressure?"

"No. How high is it?"

"210/130. Really high. We need to take you to the ER."

"No, no, no. I can't do that. I have a very important appointment later this morning," Warner lied, his voice rising in alarm.

"Our rules say you go to the ER," said the cop. "We have no choice."

"What about my car? My appointment? What if I refuse to go?"

"You'll have to sign a release. But my advice is to go get treated. You could have a stroke or heart attack with pressure that high."

"Gimme the release and I'll sign it. Then am I free to go?"

"Yeah, you can, but not a good idea."

"Why was I pulled out of line?"

"Spot check. We do it all the time. We found nothing suspicious so you're clear in that department. But we're worried about your health."

"Gimme that release. I wanna get goin'," he said, breathing out in relief, but at the same time, concerned about his out-of-control blood pressure. He signed the paper and went to his car feeling a little better. *Must have been the stress, bet my pressure's down and okay now.* Oh crap, hope my signature was illegible enough. Gotta remember, I'm Bill Reynolds now.

He drove over the two-lane steel girder bridge and saw the Customs Shed on the Mexican side. *One more to go.*

He waited while the Mexican border police dawdled with the cars and trucks ahead. *Typical. Mexicans are in a continual state of siesta with their droopy eyelids and lethargic movement. But I'll put up with this to get outta here. Almost there.*

When he finally got to the booth, he had to wait while the overweight guard fired what Warner thought was Spanish chatter over his phone, words that Warner never understood despite growing up in Texas where Spanish was in constant use. He never thought learning this foreign language was worth doing. *They should all learn English.* When the guard finished his conversation, he turned toward Warner, glaring at him.

"Passport!" he shouted at Warner, who felt like yelling back but restrained himself in a rare display of self-control. He handed his fake passport to the guard, who scrutinized it for what seemed like an eternity. *What the hell's he looking for?* The guard looked at him, then back at the passport and sat stone still. Minutes ticked by and Warner wondered if he should pass a bribe to him. He took out a hundred- dollar bill and held it against the steering wheel and watched the guard's eyes follow his movements. The guard's head nodded slightly, and Warner passed him the bill. His passport was quickly returned, and the guard waved him through.

I wonder whether that spic knew his passport was fake or if this is standard practice for Mexican cops when an American passes through. Warner sighed as he followed signs to Carr Al Puente Internacional on his way to Ciudad Camargo and freedom. Finally, he could relax and head for his five-star mountain retreat and plan the next leg of his escape.

The car chugged up the mountain with Warner trying to push it past its meager horsepower. *This sure as hell isn't a Ferrari. I'm going to miss that red beauty. After this ordeal, I deserve to treat myself to something even better. Maybe a midnight blue Lamborghini.* He maneuvered his car into the lodge's parking area and flagged a porter from the lush entryway. He felt somewhat light-headed. *Shit, of course. The altitude. I forgot it takes a few days to adjust.*

Once in his room he unpacked his bags and went to take a shower, trying to wash off the events of the day along with the sweat. As he dried himself, sudden searing pain tore through his chest bending him over, his body crashing down on the bathroom floor, his shoulder striking the toilet adding to his agony. Breathing heavily, he dragged himself, hand over hand, to the phone, knocking it off the bedside table. He retrieved the receiver and punched the operator key.

"Send a doctor," he gasped. "I think I'm having a heart attack." He dropped the phone, and his head slumped to the carpet.

Within minutes the door swung open, and a gigantic man rushed in and slapped a blood pressure cuff onto his arm, introducing himself as a physician assistant.

"Where's your pain?" he asked calmly.

"Right under my breastbone," Warner replied. "And down my left arm."

"You gotta go to the hospital, Mr. Reynolds," the PA said. "Your blood pressure is way up and your symptoms tell me you're having serious heart problems."

Warner considered the consequences of being admitted to a hospital in Mexico. *I could pay cash, I have plenty on me, but I shouldn't be in a public place. But if I don't go, I could die.*

"I'm American. Will they take cash?" he asked.

"No problem. They always welcome cash. I'll arrange an ambulance. They'll want cash too."

Waiting for the ambulance to arrive he had another episode of searing pain in his chest. The PA gave him intravenous morphine and he floated off into a semiconscious state. When he woke up, he was in an ICU attached to monitors. A fresh-faced Mexican nurse smiled at him. Her rapid fire Spanish irritated Warner.

"I only speak English," he growled at her.

She apologized and switched immediately to American English.

"You're in St Maria Hospital, in stable condition. Your ECG shows you've had a blockage in the blood-flow to your heart resulting in a patch of heart muscle being damaged. Are you in pain now?"

"A little, in my left arm." As he said this, his face screwed up in another wave of pain. "And in my chest."

The nurse adjusted the flow of pain meds in his IV. Again, he lapsed into unconsciousness. His ECG reflected this new compromise, and the nurse hurriedly obtained a new blood sample and called for the doctor. When they arrived, they found the ECG now showing ventricular fibrillation and began resuscitation. Within minutes the ECG showed a flat line. Reginald Warner, AKA Bill Reynolds, was dead.

Chapter 43

Dear Mom,

I love this place! Once we got through all the classes on social distancing, wearing of masks, handwashing and sanitizing, things have settled down. It's so cool, and my roommate is a perfect fit. She's from Philadelphia, majoring in Classics (who does that?), loves the same music I do, and likes to jog. We go together a lot. Classes are good so far but only about half the kids can go due to space limitations. Everyone else get lectures online and we alternate. I like to go and listen and talk to the instructor. She's so cool.

How are you guys? Give George a hug from me! So glad you've found each other. I'm content right now not to have a boyfriend, I'm so busy getting used to being here. Love,

Debbie

Glad she's happy and safe, Dina thought. Ever since Warner's night visit that culminated in the dog shooting and his dramatic escape, Dina couldn't sleep, even though he'd been caught, tried and convicted, and so had a lot of the management group from Pylea. *If only Warner were behind bars, I'd feel a lot better.* As long as he's walking around free before his sentencing, he was an existential threat. And now she fully understood what everyone had warned her about when they warned her about what she was doing at Pylea.

Dina hadn't sought another job yet, not feeling confident about her judgment since taking the job at Pylea. Her anxiety was amplified by having nothing to occupy her mind while George was at work and Deb was at college. He called her a couple of times each day, but she still felt threatened that Warner or some of his henchmen might try to exact revenge for her part in exposing Pylea.

She started when she heard a key turn in the door but was relieved when George strode through the door with a broad smile.

"I have some interesting news," he said. "Our friend Reginald Warner died in a Mexican hospital yesterday."

"Died? In Mexico?" Dina's eyes brightened and her mouth literally dropped open.

"I heard from our prosecutor friends, furious when he skipped bail, that Mexican police had notified them that a man identified as Bill Reynolds died in a local hospital of a coronary," George said. "Turns out his passport and wallet identification papers were discrepant. In his wallet was a Massachusetts Driver's License with his real name on it. Pretty dumb of him not to get that changed when he got his fabricated passport. From there they found he was on a US national list of bail jumpers, so they contacted prosecutors here. What do you think of that?"

Dina sat down on the sofa, head in hands, sobbing. George moved next to her and put his arm around her shoulders, surprised at her reaction.

"You knew he jumped bail? Why didn't you tell me?" Dina asked through her tears.

"You were worried enough. I had someone watching our house to make sure you were safe. It was more likely he'd leave as soon as he could. You should be happy he's out of our lives. What's the matter?"

"I...I am happy," she stammered, "that's why I'm crying, you big dope. I'm so relieved."

George laughed in his deep baritone.

"I'll never understand women," he chuckled. "Let's let Deb know so she can cry too."

Chapter 44

Tom settled on genitourinary conditions as his new specialty since trauma surgery was not an option for robotic surgery. He met with engineers from the manufacturer of a robot model the company was modifying to serve his peculiar circumstance. There were several possibilities. One was to fit the left arm port with an adapter for his mouth, allowing him to use movements of his lips and teeth to perform what a functional left hand would do. Another was adapting a foot pedal for his bare left foot, using it to manipulate the left arm in the robotic tower over the patient.

He tried both mock-up models and found the foot pedal was easier than the mouth-operated arm. Tom was encouraged with even that modicum of success. *Reminds me of that movie with Daniel Day-Lewis called My Left Foot.* After a couple of weeks, the engineers had a test model that he practiced with compulsively. He became adept in coaxing his foot to maneuver the left robotic arm to accomplish tasks an ordinary surgeon would perform with his left arm.

"Cyn, it's so much fun to manipulate this gadget. I think it's even more precise than when I was operating in a conventional way. And my foot is more versatile than I ever thought it could be," he said as they stir-fried a shrimp and vegetable combo for dinner.

"You know," Cynthia said, "they're training nurses to work in robotic operating theaters with young residents learning how to run those machines from their first days of residency. Pretty avant-garde stuff."

"How're our wedding plans going?" Tom asked, knowing that Cynthia was preoccupied with this. He didn't want enthusiasm about his new passion to crowd out talking about their November wedding. Over dinner they had a spirited and light-hearted discussion about the wedding, the invitation list that had surpassed two hundred, and the non-denominational service itself. Their honeymoon had been set for Barbados. Bermuda weather in December would be too cool.

"Did you hear the news about Warner?" Tom asked in his off-hand way.

"No, now what did that miscreant do?"

"He's dead. Died of a heart attack in Mexico."

"Holy cow! Are you kidding? How'd he get there?"

He told her the complete tale of his skipping bail and ending up, literally, in a Mexican hospital.

"Well, I can't weep bitter tears over that wretched man. Does Dina know?"

"Oh yeah, George told me today, so she knows by now."

"Who gets the million-dollar bail money?"

"The state. How do you suppose that will that be spent?"

"Is it sacrilegious to raise a glass in celebration of his passing?" Cynthia asked.

"My mother's not here, so I'll toast to that!" Tom said as they clinked glasses.

"Another thing to celebrate is the congressional hearing on Brill-Rafferty," he said. "Your testimony, along with that of Hannah, Barbara Simon, and Norman Wise made a big impression. I'm optimistic that new law will rise out of that."

Cynthia looked at her humble fiancé. "I knew you'd never take credit for positively impacting the healthcare of the country, but you were definitely the catalyst."

Of course, Tom blushed in response to her remark. "Actually," he said, "it feels pretty damn good to be so close to accomplishing what we set out to do." And Cynthia was gifted with one of Tom's most charming smiles.

Chapter 45

"Senator Blake, I'm watching your committee's hearings on the Blair-Rafferty bill. Kill it or be killed. It's bad law," the email message said.

On his website was posted a similar message. "A friend from a drug industry political action committee told me they're gonna ad blitz any legislation stifling their industry. Better watch out!"

He got a recording on his Senate phone: "Kill Blair-Rafferty or you'll pay for it in more ways than one!" The message ended with a string of profanity.

Blake had been a senator for three terms and had confronted anger before, but what he was hearing now was several decibels higher. Threats of political retribution were one thing, but now threats to his life were coming in. He heard that the chairs of the HELP and judiciary committees, also holding hearings on Brill-Rafferty, were getting similar threatening messages. All three had promised Rafferty they would press on despite threats. What else could they do?

The hearings wound down with testimony from deputies from federal agencies who advocated for the proposed law because of tax-saving implications, especially the language about Medicare negotiations with drug makers. The patent office commissioner said she had seen numerous examples of patent extensions based on minor changes in drug chemistry or dosage changes and her agency would welcome changes to restrict using patent laws. The FDA witness saw ways in which his agency could draft regulations to address legal importation of medications reducing costs to US consumers. The FDA saw these as positive improvements but made a pitch for more funding to support added administrative burdens.

Senator Blake sent the bill to the full senate for a vote where it comfortably passed, drawing yeas and nays along usual partisan lines. After conference committee review, it would go to the president. Blake expected his signature promptly. He knew there'd be legal challenges, but he'd done his job and hoped the courts would do theirs.

A 77-year-old widower, Blake lived alone in a small apartment near Du Pont Circle. He'd had it since he came to Washington twenty years ago. Paul, his regular Uber driver, drove him home most evenings. They bonded around the Nationals during baseball season and the Wizards basketball team during winter. Tonight, after the legislation passed, they arrived at his apartment tired but happy. His long career in Washington had its ups and downs, but these hearings had been nerve-wracking but gratifying. He felt he'd conducted them honorably and fairly.

Disentangling his legs from under the front seat, Blake gave Paul his usual twenty-dollar tip and climbed out. He stumbled slightly as he lugged his heavy briefcase to the brick building's entrance. Paul always waited at the curb until he was sure the Senator got into the foyer. As he watched the Senator fumbling to get his keys out, he noticed movement in the shrubbery beside the door. Focusing his attention on Blake, he jumped out of the car as a figure emerged from the bushes. The person lunged toward the elderly senator, wrestling him to the ground. Paul dashed to help, jumping a small bald man as he thrusted a knife toward Blake's neck. Paul and the assailant tussled on the ground as a stunned Blake grabbed his phone and dialed 911.

"Need help fast. A thug is trying to kill me! My driver is fighting him."

The dispatcher radioed cruisers in DuPont Circle to respond immediately to the address. Blake wanted to smash the attacker with his briefcase, but the two men were rolling around on the ground. He didn't want to disable Paul by mistake. At last Paul dislodged the knife from the perpetrator's hand. Blake seized it as it spun across the walk, tossing it into the bushes. As sirens announced approaching police cars, Paul and the aggressor were still grappling on the ground. When the police arrived, Blake gasped "The man in the orange sweatshirt is Paul, my driver. That other guy tried to kill me. Paul saved my life."

"On your feet with your hands up," the officer shouted. Paul shoved the man away from him and got to his feet. The assailant lay on the ground, hands over his head, subdued. One of the cops handcuffed him and forced him into the cruiser. The other cop took statements from Paul and Blake. When the police departed, Blake invited Paul into his apartment to decompress and share a beer.

"Senator Blake Attacked with a Knife at Home" the morning headline broadcasted followed by a tsunami of attention from local and national news media. *"Assailant being questioned but no information available."*

Talking heads on television were outraged, they were "shocked" by the attack and speculated endlessly on motive. Was this a terrorist attack or a random assault?

Questions abounded about the attacker's background. Spokespersons from both political parties decried the incident and urgently called for increased security for members of congress. The FBI joined local law enforcement to determine whether this was an individual act, a conspiracy or a terrorist act.

***

Reading about Blake's close confrontation with death made Tom's heart pound, not just from anger but also from lurid recall of his own near fatal beating. Beads of sweat covered his forehead as he read how an alert driver's care for the senator rescued him from certain death. Had he not lingered to watch while the aging senator entered his apartment, the senator would certainly have been stabbed to death.

What possible gain could there be in killing an elderly senator at this point after the bill had been signed into law by the president? This must be a warning shot marking a first in this new but different kind of drug war, a pushback to laws limiting profit from drug sales. Would there be other assailants attacking other congressmen and women? What about his PharmaTruth employees and board members? What action should he take to protect them? Would other advocacy groups also face these new threats?

"George, heard the news about Senator Blake?" Tom said on his phone.

"I did. I told you, what you're doing is sure to piss some people off. And they're playing real hardball with big bucks at stake," George said. "We gotta be careful and stay alert for every little signal. We need to train our staff to pay attention to everything around them. I'll organize some training sessions."

"I'll call a staff meeting today. Can you be there around four?"

"Of course. I'll get going on a presentation."

Tom thought of others who could be in the crosshairs: Cynthia, Norman Wise, Hannah Dorst, Barbara Simon, Gwen Owen. This threat of bodily harm prompted a wave of light-headedness to come over Tom. He started sweating and had to remember Dr. Lyon's strategies to rein in having his PTSD trigger a full-on panic attack.

"Cyn, we're having a staff meeting at 4 o'clock to advise on safety in light of the attack on Senator Blake's life. Can you come?"

"Relieved you're doing this. I'll be there. Are you okay? You sound tense."

"Truthfully, I'm on slightly shaky ground, worrying about putting people that I encouraged to testify in danger. Is someone's life worth challenging an entrenched system?"

"What's your answer to that?" Cynthia asked.

"I want to believe that everyone who participated in the hearings understood the risk. But did I state that strongly enough? Or did I want to get this bill passed so much that I underplayed the risks?"

"Tom, so many lives are going to be better because of being able to get the medicine they need. As far as I'm concerned, it was worth it. Even though I feel a little scared. But you're addressing that with this meeting, right?"

"That's the intention. Thanks, Cyn. Guess it was expected, like George said."

"I'll see you later, and Tom, I'm so glad you felt comfortable telling me you were nervous. We've come a long way. Love you."

"Love you, too," Tom said. And knowing that she was his future partner cheered him up and grounded him for the other calls he had to make.

****

"Norman, please call me at your earliest convenience," Tom told Wise's message recorder. Within minutes he returned the call.

"I know why you're calling. I heard about Senator Blake. Scary stuff," Wise said.

"Have you been threatened?"

"No, but I think I'm being followed. I see the same car day after day sitting down the street from my house. It's not one of the neighbors' cars, I recognize all of them. I told the local police. They said they'd check it out, but I've heard nothing back. Any advice?"

"We're having a staff meeting at four this afternoon. George Logan, our chief of security, will talk to staff about personal safety, what precautions each of them should take, how and when they should report their fears and suspicions, when to ask for police help, etcetera. You're welcome to join us. I'll tell our front desk downstairs."

"I'll come. I knew I'd get blowback from my testimony. I worried about personal verbal attacks but repressed thoughts of actual physical encounters. Now I'm worried."

"See you this afternoon," Tom said.

Tom called Hannah Dorst and arranged with Max and Casey to pick her up and bring her to the office for the briefing.

"Now don't you worry, Hannah, we'll be sure you're looked after," Tom told her.

His last call was to Dr. Lyon. He needed a therapy session for himself.

***

Congresswoman Eva Brill had a military background and was no stranger to violence, but the attack on Senator Blake unnerved her. This was supposed to be a civil society, and this kind of attack went against the personal safety she believed should surround everyone's daily lives, despite frequent reports of school, church, synagogue and theater shootings. *Am I next on the list? Who did this? Could the drug industry be this craven? That's hard to believe, but there must be a connection between signing the bill that bore our names and the attack on Blake.*

She lived in Georgetown and called her local police.

"This is Congresswoman Brill. I live on Reservoir Rd Northwest in Georgetown. I need to talk to the Desk Sergeant about police protection." Brill knew she'd better call a staff meeting to reassure them and advise her team about personal safety. She knew they were all edgy.

***

Police questioned the assailant, a 38-year-old white man named Leroy Tate who had a record of eight previous arrests for assault, drug possession and disorderly conduct.

He scoffed when they asked him if he were a member of any political party or movement.

"Politics sucks. I live in the real world, ya know. I needed money bad and a guy I recognized at this bar I go to, we were talkin,' and I asked him if he could lend me some money. He showed me $1000 cash. Said if I'd kill some old dude, it'd be mine. Told me where this guy lived, what he looked like. He even showed me his picture. Told me he usually got to his apartment seven-thirty, eight o'clock. I never was a hit man before but guess that guy had the feeling I needed dough bad. Gave me $100 down payment."

"How were you gonna get the rest of the money?"

"Told me he'd meet me in Rock Creek Park."

"And you trusted him?"

"No choice."

"He tell you why he wanted him dead?"

"Nah, not a word. I didn't ask either. Didn't matter to me."

"You know Mr. Blake is a United States senator?"

"You shitting me? A senator? Oh Christ, I'm in real trouble now."

"We're calling the public defender's office, get you a lawyer."

Over the next days, Tate described the man in the bar as white, in his thirties, medium height, balding, beardless, wearing a blazer, khakis and sneakers with no socks. The cops went to the bar to question the bartender who was working when Tate said the deal went down. He remembered Tate, a frequent customer, but couldn't recall the other man.

"Think about it some more. We'll be back. We're looking for this guy because he was behind the attack on Senator Blake."

"Jesus H. Christ. I'll rack my brain and try to help, honestly," the bartender said.

The cops looked at each other trying not to betray skepticism. They knew from experience finding this mysterious briber was a fool's errand. Tate's description of him could fit thousands of guys walking around Washington DC any day of the year.

Chapter 46

Pylea was in shambles after Warner and the board members were convicted. Tom thought of Ahmed. Entrusting the manufacturing of his life-saving antibiotic to Warner was a disastrous decision that must be depressing.

Huh. Wonder if I could recruit a venture capital group to rescue Pylea and get Ahmed back into the process?

"Ahmed, this is Tom Barrett. I'm calling to touch base. Give me a call."

He called his board member, Elizabeth Stuckey, at Associated Industries in Atlanta. Tom admired her contributions at board meetings and knew she was well connected to business communities in Atlanta as well as nationally and internationally.

"Elizabeth, I'm sure you've followed the plight of Pylea. What you may not have heard is that Reginald Warner, Pylea's CEO, was found dead in a Mexican hotel recently, having skipped bail to escape sentencing in Massachusetts. The company's in receivership and for sale. Think we could round up some venture capitalists to buy it? The antibiotic is an outstanding medication. I know the fellow who invented it, Ahmed Mohammed, works at Hempstead Institute. Give me a call when you have time."

A few hours later Ahmed called.

"Tom, so good to hear from you. What're you doing these days?"

"I'm flyin' high Ahmed. I'm learning how to be a surgeon again."

"What do you mean?"

"I'm learning robotic surgery. It's amazing. The engineers who designed the robot are fitting it with a loop that allows my left foot to guide the left robotic arm. I move my foot to the left and the arm moves to the left. I lift my foot and up goes the arm. My right hand does most of the work, as it always did when I did conventional surgery, but now it's as though I have my left hand back. I didn't believe this could work until I tried it, but it's going great!"

"That's so cool! I know how much you loved surgery. What a terrific idea."

Tom took a deep breath to calm his enthusiasm.

"But I didn't call about that. I called about Pylea. I called one of our board members who might get a group of business associates to buy the company. I wanted to give you hope your antibiotic might still find its way into use."

"Oh, that would be a gift from Allah. Pylea has been such a disaster. I should have trusted my gut about Warner early on, but I was so eager to get the drug deployed," he lamented. "What do you think the chances are?"

"Don't know. Our board member is well-connected, and the drug is sure to be a winner. We can hope that it'll work out, but I'll let you know when I hear back from Ms. Stuckey," Tom said. "So, how're things at Hempstead?"

"Well, only so-so. We're having problems with funding. Not unusual, we're a small non-profit and not doing sexy stuff in research, you know, like immunotherapy and CRISPR. So, it's a little anxiety-producing not knowing which way the wind's blowing. My grants run out in about six months and after that I'm not sure what I'm going to do."

"That's all the more reason to get someone to buy Pylea. You'd be an ideal person to head it up."

"Whoa, not sure about that. I made a big mistake trusting Warner. People in business might question my judgment. And I have little administrative experience."

"Your judgment is fine. Just because an unscrupulous man misled you doesn't mean you have poor judgment. And you could surround yourself with competent good people to help with administration. You know how important teamwork is."

"Well, I'm interested in getting Cidal into the hands of doctors. But not at the price Warner was setting, nowhere near that. It could be done for much, much less. It's easy to produce."

"I'll call back when I know more."

"Thanks Tom. And I'm happy to know about your success with robotics. Plus, I hear you're getting married."

"Boy, news travels fast. Well, you're on the invitation list, but I hope I don't have to wait until the wedding to see you."

***

Dina picked up her mail at her old address and was sorting through the catalogs and coupons, laughing at the offers of fantastic products never seen by human eyes. Some first-class mail was mixed in with the dross, but one letter struck her eye. It was from Horace Finley, Attorney-At-Law, Dallas Texas. *Who can that be?* She turned the envelope over, looking for the postmark. Back at George's condo, she sat at her small desk and slit open the envelope.

Dear Ms. Robbins,
I represent Reginald Warner.

Dina's heart plummeted. *He's after me from the grave.*

As you may know, my client died recently. I am his executor and have been his personal lawyer for many years. A few months ago, at his instruction, I wrote a new will. It is a simple will that has been through Probate Court.

In it he leaves all his earthly possessions to you. He has no living relatives. This includes personal property both in Texas and in Cambridge Massachusetts, and his bank accounts. His personal bank account in Massachusetts has a few thousand dollars and he had an account in Grand Cayman. The approximate balance in that account is $11,769,234.34.

His personal property here in Texas is a small parcel of land near his birthplace. I await your instruction about how you'd like to handle this. I can put it into the hands of a realtor here and when it sells send you the proceeds. I've terminated his condo lease in Cambridge so there is no need for action on your part related to that. If you authorize me, I can arrange for his personal effects in Cambridge to be sold and send you the proceeds for that as well.

Contact me at your earliest convenience with a wire transfer number for your bank account and I will carry out Mr. Warner's instructions.

Sincerely,
   Horace Finley, JD
   Dallas, Texas

Dina read the letter over and over, astonished.

When exactly did he write this will? And why didn't he change it after I betrayed him? Maybe he wrote it in a drunken fog early in our relationship and then had no recollection after he sobered up? Oh my God, inheriting almost $12 million dollars from a man I detested, who I was instrumental in bringing down, is beyond ironic. Could there be a mistake? Maybe it's a hoax? Some kind of scam?

She couldn't wait until George got home to talk about this over a strong drink.

Around seven, later than usual, having run the conference at the office on safety, George was back. He made a beeline for his favorite chair, slumped down and exhaled a long sigh.

"You must have heard that Senator Blake's life was threatened yesterday," George said before Dina had a chance to say hello. "I had to run a conference at the office to educate and reassure the staff. A lot of people are nervous."

"Yeah, I did hear about that. The senator's okay, right? And they caught the guy?"

"Yes, and yes. But no information about who might be behind the attack. The assailant was a hired killer, but an amateur, very inept. He says some guy in a bar gave him money to go after Blake, says he didn't even know he was a senator, so he's a real ignoramus.

"So, what's new with you? You look funny," George said, finally noticing Dina's expression.

"Well, got this letter," Dina said, holding it up. "Look it over and see what you think."

George took it from Dina, looked at the envelope, and read the letter. As he absorbed its content, his eyebrows rose, and his mouth dropped open.

"Good Lord, this is incredible. He must have written this when he thought you were the love of his life. Must have thought he was gonna spend the rest of his life in bliss. Can't fault him for that logic," George said, winking at her.

Dina smiled. "Well, he had to have done it when he was drunk. If it's legitimate. How can we know?"

"I'll run a check on Mr. Horace Finley, see what this cat's all about. It's a downtown Dallas address, so it seems real. Should I do this now or after we eat something? Oh, never mind, I'll do it now," George said, seeing Dina's forehead crease with frown-lines, her mouth draw down and her hands at her temples.

"Thank you. I'll throw some pasta together while you do that. Pesto or Bolognese sauce?"

"Pesto. This shouldn't take too long." He went to his computer. After a few clicks, he went to the kitchen.

"Okay, got several takes on Finley. He's an expensive downtown Dallas lawyer with credentials to choke a pig. He's definitely legit. Tomorrow, you should contact him by phone and get the rest of the story.

"I was gonna ask you to marry me but now you'd think I'm doing that for your money," George said, laughing.

"I accept! And if you back out when I find out there's a big mistake about this inheritance, I'll probably have to kill you," Dina said.

There was a moment when they looked at each other, realizing what had just been spoken. Then they collapsed in a fit of hilarity.

Chapter 47

Elizabeth Stuckey was in constant motion after Tom's call. Atlanta was a hotbed of venture capitalists, and she knew many of them.

"Tom, I've got a great lead on several venture capitalists here in Atlanta who seem interested in Pylea. I think we'll be able to swing this. Maybe could use a few million more depending on what the receiver is asking. When's the sale?"

"Not sure of that. But good work. Soon as I know I'll be in touch."

"Perfect. I'll let you know when the investors are firmly committed."

***

George, still reeling from the news about Warner's will, found Tom in his office, staring out the window.

"Where's your mind, my friend?" George asked.

"In my robot chamber," he replied.

"You're really into that creepy high-tech stuff. Next thing we know you're gonna buy a Watson for the office and replace all the people with AI."

"I'm only into robotic surgery, not the rest of it," Tom chuckled. "But, George, I'm telling you, I'm so in love with my robot, I can't tell you how much it's changing my outlook."

Tom shifted into a moment that could only be characterized as an absence from current reality. If he'd had an EEG running, he would probably record a change in brain waves, showing only alpha rhythm. He stopped talking and gazed out the window, leaving George and PharmaTruth in the distance.

"George, I'm thinking about doing robotic surgery full time when I finish my fellowship. I believe strongly in the mission of PharmaTruth, so I'm torn. My first love has always been surgery. I don't know what to do. What do you think?"

George's familiarity with the workings of Tom's mind began when they were fellow patients and then amateur sleuths at Zylinski. George's remarkable insight had grown as their relationship at PharmaTruth had matured. He'd lately been aware of Tom's gradual drift away from passion with the PharmaTruth mission since his romance with robotic surgery. He'd anticipated this question. Tom had been increasingly absent from his office, having his affair with Ms. DaVinci, the robot.

"Have you talked about this with Cyn?" George asked.

"She knows how much I'm enjoying the fellowship, but I've been reluctant to broach the subject of doing it full time. I should talk to her, but I thought I'd run it by you first. You've been my best friend for a long time and through some, shall we say, interesting times."

"Well, it seems to me your heart is telling you what to do. As the saying goes, follow your bliss."

"But everyone depends on me here. I can't let everyone down by just doing what I want for myself." He sighed.

"My daddy told me that whenever you think you're essential, put your finger in a glass of water, take it out and see what kind of a hole it makes," George said. "People die, get sick, move on all the time. No one's indispensable, even though it's hard on the old ego to consider that someone else can do your job as well as you, maybe even better, but it's a fact of life."

"You know, you should have been a psychologist. This isn't the first time I've asked, how'd you get so damned wise?"

"Come off it, I'm only telling you what's common sense. None of us can see things clearly when we're in the center of the ring."

"Who do you think should be in charge here if I leave? You interested?"

"You kidding? Not my cup of tea. I like what I do here and hope to continue under any leadership, but I have no illusions about running a non-profit. How about your guy Burseik? He seems like a smart dude, used to sorting out issues, a good and likable leader."

"He'd be good, you're right. There are probably others we know about and some we don't know about. The board would have to do a search."

"Let me tell you some interesting news," George said, looking at Tom over his steel-rimmed glasses. "Dina is rich."

"How so? Because she's got you around?"

"Well, that, of course," he laughed. "But she inherited a bunch of money."

"Who from? I know her mother died, the reason for her interest in Pylea, but that was some time ago."

"You'd never guess, so I'll tell you. She was in Warner's will. She got a letter from his lawyer. He told her there was over twelve million dollars in a Cayman account he left her in his will."

"No shit? What the hell? Now I've heard everything. I'm flabbergasted."

"Now we got to figure out what to do with it."

Tom's eyes lit up. "I have an idea."

"Uh-oh. I can smell trouble here. What?"

"Go in with a group of investors to buy Pylea. Liz Stuckey is sounding out this bunch of venture capitalists. Maybe Dina would be interested in being part of that. Remember, she signed on at Pylea to help market Cidal because her mother died from a resistant organism. Wouldn't that be poetic justice?"

George looked out the window, marveling at the way the world worked.

"I'll run it by her. It's worth considering."

***

"Liz Stuckey here. Consider me a great success," she bragged. "I have four VC's who want to go with others to buy Pylea. How's that for quick results?"

"Well, I always knew VCs were impetuous rich people, but that's fast track squared. I have another possible investor here in Boston. I'll put her in touch with you if she wants to join them. Great work Liz. Thanks."

"The next step is due diligence looking into financial details with the receiver. I'll take care of that and then let you know what else needs to happen."

This added impetus to Tom's decision to loosen his role at PharmaTruth. His understanding of the business aspects of running a non-profit was minimal at best and he had little interest in mastering it. The smell of an operating room, the allure of caring for patients and the seduction of learning new technology were attracting him like a bright blossom draws a butterfly. He needed a smooth exit strategy.

***

"Tom, this is Dina. George told me about your brainstorm. I'd like to know more about this. What can you tell me?"

"I just got off a call from Liz Stuckey. She has four venture capitalists interested in buying Pylea. I think you ought to talk to her. I'm not of much use in this kind of thing but she is," Tom told her. "If you join this group, well, I may be getting ahead of myself on this, but anyhow, one thing I'd like you to consider is hiring Ahmed Mohammed. You know, the pharmacologist who discovered Cidal. I think he'd be a natural as leader of the company that produces and sells this medicine. He is squeaky clean ethically and a brilliant guy. He's also a gem of a person."

"Wow, Tom, you *are* getting way ahead of me. I'm still working on getting my mind used to this inheritance thing. Nothing prepared me for this, you know. I'm really bewildered and scared," Dina said in a tremulous voice. "Can you tell me who the hell Liz Stuckey is?"

"Sorry Dina, I don't mean to come on so strong, but this is so exciting. Liz is on our board at PharmaTruth. She's the head of Associated Industries, a group of business leaders in Atlanta. I've found her to be a great resource and a dedicated board member." He gave her phone number and email address to Dina. "Give her a call. I told her about the possibility of another investor; she'll be expecting your call."

Later, Tom felt guilty about pushing Dina so hard, but he rationalized his behavior by blaming his surgical personality, sometimes impetuous but well-meaning. He hoped her conversation with Liz would go well.

Chapter 48

Tom, Cynthia, George and Dina considered a double wedding but there were complications. Tom and Cynthia wanted a church wedding with organ music, so they chose a traditional service; George grew up Baptist and Dina was Jewish. They compromised with a Unitarian service.

"George, what's your wedding date?" Tom asked when George answered his phone.

"January fourteenth, ten o'clock at the Arlington Street Church downtown. We're having a rather small wedding with the reception downstairs. Have maybe fifty people coming, including you and Cynthia. Remember Matt from Zylinski? I tracked him down and he'll be there. Most of the other people you won't know, people from my hometown and some of Dina's friends. Of course, Deb will be there as the maid of honor."

"Our wedding is a month before that," Tom said. "Glad of that since I want you to be my best man. Can you do that?"

"I'd be honored to be your best man. How about returning the favor? Will you be back from your honeymoon by the fourteenth?"

"Yep. Deal."

Both men got lost in their private thoughts as they contemplated this major life change into a married state.

"You still there?" George asked.

"Yup. I'm curious to know what Dina's thinking is about that group that wants to buy Pylea. I know I'm prying, but my curiosity gets the better of me."

"She talked to the Stuckey woman, liked her a lot. Think she's inclined to join the group. I'm skeptical, but I always am about that industry. I know too much bad stuff about them. She told me about your idea about Ahmed. That's the best part."

"He'll be at my wedding, along with Akira and Alicia, and a bunch of others from Zylinski. It'll be a great reunion. The one guy I couldn't invite was that prick Deitrich."

"Oh, your best buddy who called security on you, because you tried to assault him. Can't imagine why you're not inviting him!" George chided Tom.

"Okay, okay, smartass. But you'll be able to see a lot of our old friends from those dark days. By the way, you still on nepenthe?"

"Oh, yeah, wouldn't leave home without it. How 'bout you?"

"Likewise. Still in counseling too. Saw Dr. Lyon the other day. That attack on Senator Blake got my engine running funny, but I'm okay. Lyon is so skilled. I always feel better after my time with him.

"Keep me posted on the Stuckey-Dina conversation. Tell Dina she can call me anytime. Take care," Tom said, signing off.

***

A few days later the conference room at PharmaTruth was jammed. Everyone who worked there was asked to come to an important meeting called by Dr. Barrett. No one knew what it was about. Most thought it was about the Brill-Rafferty bill and the attack on Senator Blake. After everyone found a place to stand or sit, Tom stood up at a podium, an unusual event as he usually spoke more informally.

"I asked you her for several reasons," Tom said. "First, and most important, Brill-Rafferty is now law." Applause flooded the room, with whoops and hollers from staff and board members alike. "That means our efforts have borne fruit and thanks go to all of you for your part in bringing this about. Margaret Mead said 'Never underestimate the ability of a small group of committed individuals to change the world. Indeed, they are the only ones who ever have.' You have proven the truth of that statement.

"But don't forget this task has only just begun. This is a tributary leading to a river of needs. The mission of PharmaTruth will continue to be keeping big pharma's feet to the fire, and that mission won't be accomplished until every man, woman and child can get medicines they need at a price they can afford.

"The next item on my agenda is hard for me," Tom said, avoiding eye contact with any of the people who had worked so passionately with him since PharmaTruth was founded.

"As many of you know, I'm a surgeon to my core. Not being able to practice my calling has been a hole in my life. Recently an innovative technology, robotic surgery, has offered me a new opportunity to go back into the operating room. I've recently started a fellowship learning how a robotic surgical model can substitute for my left arm. I can't tell you how grateful I am this ingenious instrument has enabled me to return to the work I love. Over the next year

I'll be transitioning from being CEO of PharmaTruth to the life of a practicing surgeon again."

Groans and shouts of "no" echoed through the conference room. When they died down, Tom's blush faded, and he brushed a tear from his cheek.

"I really dreaded announcing this because everyone here is dear to me. I appreciate the dedication and hard work you've all brought to our organization. Getting Brill-Rafferty passed is a marvel, but also important to me is the feeling of family this place has."

Tom waited a moment to gather his emotions.

"I'll be an ex-officio board member, and I promise you I'll be around. You're not rid of me, not by a long shot. In the next few weeks, we'll talk more about my successor and what lies ahead. But rest assured you'll be in good hands.

"Wendell Berry in his book "The Memory of Old Jack" wrote, 'He saw that he would be distinguished not by what he was or anything that he might become, but by what he served.'

"I think what we serve here will have lasting consequence for millions of people. Keep on keepin' on."

Epilogue

Reed Burseik took over PharmaTruth, and George continued looking after the safety of those who sought to end pharmaceutical industry corruption. Evidence from street surveillance cameras provided a new lead for discovering who was behind the attempted murder of Senator Blake, who decided to retire, not because of the assassination attempt, but because passage of Brill-Rafferty was such a meaningful accomplishment and a cap to a long and distinguished career.

Due to Pylea's complicated corporate structure, it took a long time, but ultimately the group of venture capitalists, including Dina Robbins, created a new company called T-Cidal from the ashes of Pylea. Ahmed Mohammed, the discoverer of the unique antibiotic Cidal, was unanimously selected CEO by the new T-Cidal Board of Directors. The price of a Cidal intravenous four-day inpatient treatment was under $25,000 including the paraphernalia for its administration. Congresswoman Brill and Senators Rafferty and Blake attended the announcement ceremony with Dr. Tom Barrett, who gave the keynote speech.

Acknowledgments

Friends, family and colleagues have been great sources of encouragement and advice as I wrote this novel, a sequel to *Double Blind Double Cross*. Thanks go to many: Tracy Hart, my editor, whose advice in development and refinement was critical; to my wife Betsy, whose careful readings caught mistakes in several versions of the manuscript; to friends Martha Coakley, Tom Kirkman, and Richard Cohen who gave me advice about legal aspects of the story; to Carl Heilman and Gino Carpanito for their advice on robotic surgery; to pharmacist Jeff Gonneville for valuable advice about medications; to readers Dr. Abdollah Sadeghi-Nejad, Ray Byrne, Dr. Robert Block, Jane Long, Maria Moniz, Pauli Pendleton, Mary White and Dr. Lew Stern for their suggestions; to fellow pediatrician, friend and author Dr. Stephanie Deutsch Salim for her valuable advice; to Steve Manchester for his unfailing support; to Michael Grossman for his counsel at all stages of the book's gestation; and to Kathryn Galán at Wynnpix Productions for her patience and valued advice.

Special thanks to Tom Tafuri for his excellent cover design, which captures the essence of the problems the book addresses.

About the Author

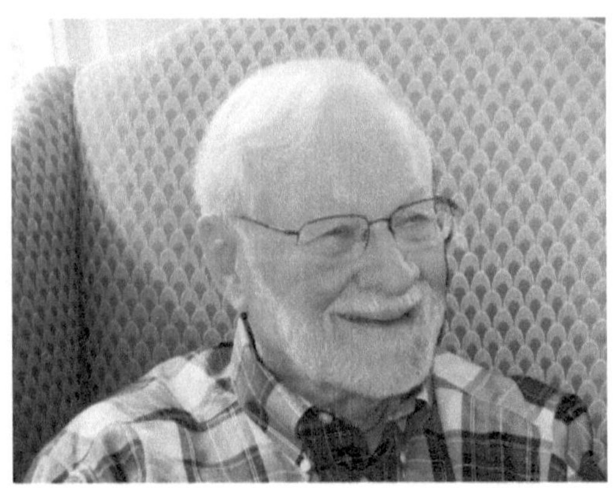

Robert M. Reece practiced, taught, and did research in pediatrics for over forty years, specializing in diagnosis and treatment of child abuse cases. He published nine textbooks, nearly fifty articles, and twenty-seven book chapters. He founded and was Editor of *The Quarterly Update* from 1993 until 2017.

His debut novel, *To Tell The Truth,* describes a fictional case of a young babysitter charged with the murder of a seven-month-old infant in her care.

In *Double Blind Double Cross,* he writes about surgeon Tom Barrett, a victim of post-traumatic stress disorder, (PTSD) and his experiences while participating in a clinical trial of a new drug for PTSD. Tom and two fellow patients immerse themselves in a high stakes investigation that reveals a shocking answer that would question practices in parts of the pharmaceutical industry.

In *Strong Medicine,* Dr. Barrett returns to shine a bright light on the pharmaceutical industry, uncovering practices that are unethical and illegal.

The Lewellyns from Vincennes is the story of a twentieth century family whose lives are buffeted by personal losses, two world wars, the Great Depression, and family triumphs. Based on a true story, its tapestry is woven with invention of scenes and fictional dialogue and is ultimately a tale of redemption and resilience.

In 2024, he published his latest novel, *About Ben,* the based-on-true story of a medical student stricken with polio who becomes the pediatrician's pediatrician.

Learn more at www.robertmreece.com